The Book on Home Hospice

Living and Dying in Comfort with Dignity

Deborah Dooler, MD CCFP (PC)

THE BOOK ON HOME HOSPICE:
LIVING AND DYING IN COMFORT WITH DIGNITY
www.HomeHospiceBook.com

Publisher
10-10-10 Publishing
Markham, ON
Canada

Contents

Dedication

I dedicate this book to my cousin, Maxine Gopsill Small, who died from cancer way too young. She faced every day with courage and laughter. She was the strongest person I have ever known. She has been an inspiration to me and is loved and missed by many.

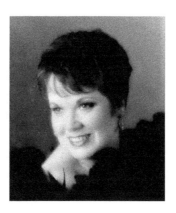

I also dedicate this book to you, the reader, and to all the people you hold near and dear. You are the true star of this book, whether a recipient of care, a caregiver, or healthcare angel. You are the everyday heroes who make this world a better, more compassionate place to be. My wish is that your journey be filled with love, light, comfort, and dignity.

Preface

I consider myself to be an old-fashioned country doctor in many ways. I come to your home with my black medical bag, I sit at your bedside, and I hold your hand and offer comfort and support in your last months, days, and hours. I laugh with you, and I cry with you, but most of all, I listen. I look into your eyes and ask how you are feeling today, and what it is that is most important to you. I want to know about your wishes and your hopes and dreams for the future. I am only a small part of the home hospice team; we are all here to support and offer hope to those who are dying, and to their families.

I see you at your best and at your worst. You don't need to get dressed for me. I will see you where you are, whether that is at the kitchen table or in bed. You are the star of the show; it is your life and your journey. I have written this book to offer you some valuable information, and share my experiences of caring for people at the end of life in their home.

It is a true privilege to be welcomed into your home. I feel truly blessed to be able to do what I am passionate about and love: to provide comfort to those in need.

My hope is that you will read this book and feel empowered to ask for and, if need be, demand that you receive home hospice care in your area. I cannot be there personally for everyone, but it is my belief that we all deserve to have access to quality home hospice care.

I send much love and blessings to you, the reader.

Dr. Deborah Dooler
Palliative Care Specialist
Award Winning Author

Foreword

The Book on Home Hospice: Living and Dying in Comfort with Dignity by Dr. Deborah Dooler is written to help you understand what it means to be diagnosed with a terminal illness. It offers practical suggestions to help you or your loved ones to manage care in your own home.

This book is an excellent resource, whether you or a loved one has been diagnosed with cancer, COPD, heart failure, ALS or any other life-limiting illness. At this difficult time in your life, *The Book on Home Hospice: Living and Dying in Comfort with Dignity* offers you valuable information on coping with a terminal illness, including managing the physical, psychological and spiritual challenges that you or your loved ones may be struggling with. It also offers you insights into the complexities and great rewards of home hospice care. You will find the book to be the most comprehensive resource on end-of-life care in the home. It can be used as a manual and journal on your journey.

Dr. Deborah Dooler is the authority on home hospice care, and she brings her vast knowledge and experience to you. Her passion for helping you to cope with trauma and loss is evident in every chapter of the book. Her book deals with death and dying in a compassionate and straightforward manner. Having met Dr. Dooler in person, I know her to be a tireless advocate for providing compassionate palliative care in the comfort of your own home.

This book contains a great deal of wisdom, and I highly recommend you read it. I found it to be an inspiration, and I am sure you will too.

Raymond Aaron
New York Times Bestselling Author

Acknowledgements

Thank you to my husband, **John Dooler,** for your unconditional love and unfailing support for everything I do. Thank you for all the hours you have spent proof reading this book; you have made it so much better than I ever dreamed it would be. I love you. You are my true soulmate.

Thank you to my children, **Rick, Amy, and Johnathon Dooler.** Having you in my life has been my one true success. I am so proud of the beautiful, loving, successful people you have become. I love you with all my heart.

I would like to offer a special thank you to my parents, **Kathy Nock** and **John Nock.** Without you, I would not be the person I am today.

I wish to say thank you to **Joan Clover** and **Alan (Bunny) Clover** for always supporting me and cheering me on. Your kind and caring nature has been an inspiration to me.

I would like to say an enormous thank you to my colleagues and friends on the **South Niagara Palliative Care Team (aka Southern Comfort):**

Sue Battersby-Campbell, NP – You are a force to be reckoned with, and I could not do it without you. You are a true expert in the field of palliative care.

Susan DeCicco – I am blessed to have you in my life. Your compassion and willingness to go above and beyond to help people is truly inspirational.

Petrusia Mulholland – You make my life so much easier. You are an amazing woman, and I am glad you are on my team.

Clarence Braun – Clare, you have been with me from day one. You carried me when I couldn't walk, and you heal my soul on a daily basis. Thank you for all you do.

Sandra Deaves – I am in awe of your compassion and resilience. Your work with children and their families has made you a perfect addition to our team.

Joanna Mataya – Thank you for your tireless efforts and support to the teams. You insulate us so we can do our work. It is greatly appreciated.

I would like to offer a special thanks to retired **Dr. Maria Becker**. You have made me a better and more mindful doctor and person. I am forever in your debt.

Thank you to Hospice Niagara, especially **Carol Nagy,** for your ongoing support and wisdom to the teams of Niagara. Thank you for advocating for better palliative care services for all. A special thanks to **Tina Van Egmond** for your contribution to Hospice in the Niagara region.

I would like to thank you, **Raymond Aaron,** for your kind forward in the book. I would like to express my gratitude to you for inspiring me to become an author. Attending your events has opened my heart and soul in a way that I never thought possible.

A special thank you to **Barbara Powers** an exceptional book architect for your kind help and wise words.

Thank you to **Jack Canfield;** you have been an inspiration to me. What I have learned from you has made me a better author and a better human being.

I would like to offer a special thank you to all the **patients and their families** who have allowed me into their lives at such a difficult and challenging time. I am inspired and awed by your love and support for what I do; thank you.

Finally, a huge thank you to all the dedicated home palliative nurses and care coordinators who are working at the bedside, providing compassionate care to offer comfort to the dying, on a daily basis:

Brenda Sinan, Cindy Perry, Colleen O'Gorman, Dawn Brown, Dennis D'Uva, Donald Aedy, Jungok Seo (Jade), Jocelyne Molnar, Kelly Karner, Kim Bradshaw, Kim Gatt, Kim

Wells, Laurie Andrychuck, Linda Serre, Meighan Truant, Nora Johnson, Paola Lawrence, Prince Gwanzura, Shari House Comeaux, Tracy Earick, Trina Lemay.

I truly admire what you do. You are true healthcare angels and a blessing to know.

Chapter 1
How You Can Use *The Book on Home Hospice: Living and Dying in Comfort with Dignity*

The act of dying is one of the acts of life.
Marcus Aurelius

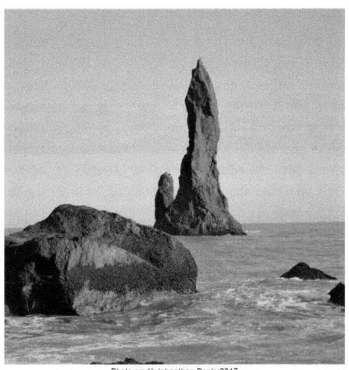

Photo.credit:Johnathon.Dooler2017

How you can benefit from *The Book on Home Hospice: Living and Dying in Comfort with Dignity*

I have written *The Book on Home Hospice: Living and Dying in Comfort with Dignity* as a resource and companion for people who may be experiencing the shock, pain, and sorrow of being diagnosed with a life-limiting, terminal illness, and for their families, caregivers, loved ones, neighbours, volunteers, and anyone else with an interest in providing comfort and dignity to those in need at the end of life. This chapter will introduce you to the structure and form of the book, and what topics will be covered in the following chapters.

The information in *The Book on Home Hospice* comes from my own personal medical practice within the hospital and community settings. As a palliative care physician, practicing, teaching, and lecturing in the Niagara Region, I have had the privilege of working with thousands of people and their families facing the end of life, over the years. I have been inspired and awestruck with the resilience and compassion of the human race. It is an inherently human trait to protect and care for the most vulnerable in our society. Death, as is birth, is a process to be shared and experienced with loved ones. It is their heroic bravery in coming to terms with their terminal illness that has inspired me to write this book. My hope is that it will help you to come to terms with the meaning of your diagnosis and help you to understand the normal process of dying, and the enormous benefits and challenges of choosing to stay in your home at the end of life. It can be one of the most rewarding and satisfying experiences for you and your loved ones, as long as the appropriate support services are in place.

As you take this journey with your family and caregivers, it can be a deeply spiritual time, full of reflection but also fear and worry about the physical and mental changes that will affect you and your whole family.

The Book on Home Hospice will help you to become familiar with the home hospice experience, as well as with those caregivers who will be in your circle of care. This includes professionals and loved ones, assisting you with planning and preparing for those practical things, such as preparing legal documents, home care set up, and safety. It will address concerns regarding the relief of common symptoms of the body: pain, breathing, energy, gastrointestinal, urinary and sexual tracts, and of the mind: depression, anxiety, confusion, agitation, and delirium. The book addresses medical emergencies, such as opioid toxicity and opioid overdose, bleeding, convulsions, superior vena cava syndrome, and spinal cord compression. As equally important to the physical and mental strains and challenges are the spiritual and religious. *The Book on Home Hospice* will discuss spirituality and religion as it pertains to you. There are suggestions for you to integrate mindfulness practice and legacy work.

The Book on Home Hospice discusses what to expect at the end of life, with an introduction to the differences between terminal sedation and medical assistance in dying. Descriptions of what to expect in the last few months, few days, and few hours are meant to educate and enlighten you with the hope to alleviate some of the fear and worry of the unknown. There will be suggestions for coping with death and what to do next. The final chapter will discuss life after death, dealing with grief and bereavement, and moving on.

The Book on Home Hospice is meant to be used as a starting point to introduce some very difficult topics of conversation. You will notice that I have provided ***Free Bonus Material at my website www.HomeHospiceBook.com** throughout the book. Please feel free to visit my website to access more detailed information as you see fit.

The Book on Home Hospice need not be read from front to back; please feel free to look at the chapters and subchapters, and choose a topic that is relevant to you at the time. Although written in a sequential way, each chapter and subchapter can stand on its own. I understand that, at times, you may be overwhelmed and exhausted; therefore, I recommend digesting the information in small bursts, or as questions may arise. There may be topics that are not pertinent to your situation—I suggest that you may want to skip these sections, with no guilt or regret. This book was written for you, and I truly hope you find it to be valuable and informative.

Citations for you

Citations can be found at the very back of *The Book on Home Hospice*; I have used the most up-to-date and relevant information available at the time of publication.

Resources for you

Throughout *The Book on Home Hospice,* you will find **some helpful definitions**. It can be challenging to navigate the world of medicine, and I hope these definitions are helpful to your understanding of the process of living with a terminal illness and dying at home.

I want you to know you are not alone, and I have provided ***Free Resources at my website www.HomeHospiceBook.com.** Please feel free to visit my website for directions on how to access resources in your location. There are many wonderful and helpful websites to visit for information on palliative care and specific disease-related associations. Please visit my website to access the most up-to-date information and links.

Special considerations for children and adolescents

Many of the suggestions in *The Book on Home Hospice* may hold true for children who are dying, but due to the complexity and specialization of dealing with the death of a child at home, it is out of the scope of this book. However, as children are an integral part of our lives and family structures, it is imperative to include them in the conversation regarding the process of dying and the death of their loved ones.

Throughout *The Book on Home Hospice,* you will find the teddy bear icon for suggestions of how to approach and support children and adolescents through their journey. It is important to introduce the idea of death, to children, as an everyday part of life; this could include discussions regarding the death of a plant or a dead bird, or the dying of a beloved pet. A child's experience with the death of a loved one can be extremely difficult, for the child and the adults around them. A child's grief can be underestimated; it may be difficult for them to express their feelings. Death can be difficult to understand at any age; and regardless of age, all children grieve.

I have added a list of resources, books, videos, and organizations that may be helpful. Throughout *The Book on Home Hospice*, there are tips and suggestions to help children understand, express, and cope with their emotions and fears. In the chapter on grief, children's bereavement responses at different developmental stages, and risk factors for complicated grieving, will be discussed.

For concerns regarding the well-being of your children, please refer to the child's family physician or pediatrician for ongoing advice. Your local hospice is an excellent resource with programs available to help families cope, as well as your local family and children's services center.

Suggestions for things you can do to bring comfort and dignity

In the last subchapter of each chapter, I have provided suggestions for you to provide comfort and dignity for either yourself or someone you care about. You will find tips on safety, symptom management, planning, and support at the end of the chapters. My hope is that they will help your experience at home to be more peaceful and comfortable.

Start the discussion about death and dying: Interesting facts about death

Did you know?
When Thomas Edison died in 1941, Henry Ford captured his dying breath in a bottle.

To start the discussion about death and dying, I have provided some interesting facts about death throughout *The Book on Home Hospice*. The purpose is to make you feel more comfortable thinking and talking about death as a natural part of life. Dying is something we human beings do continuously, not just at the end of our physical lives on this earth. [18] Every minute, 35 million of your cells die; death is not a failure of life but a part of it.

It is as natural to die as to be born.

Francis Bacon (1561-1626) British statesman and
philosopher

To make *The Book on Home Hospice* your own, I encourage you to highlight the things that are important to you, and to use this as a starting point for opening dialogue with your family, friends, and caregivers. It is through open and honest communication that you can truly begin to work through the stages and processes of living and dying, with comfort and dignity, on your own terms.

Many recent studies have shown the importance of initiating a palliative approach to care at the beginning of a terminal diagnosis, as palliative care and ongoing treatment can go hand-in-hand. Early initiation of palliative care can lead to a more comfortable and often longer life, enabling you to stay in your home and avoid hospitalizations. I have seen the effects firsthand of offering symptom relief along with psychosocial and spiritual support to relieve suffering. With symptoms resolved and stress relieved, the body is often more capable of moving through the phases of grief, from denial and anger to acceptance and peace. Unfortunately, the word palliative care, or end of life care, has many negative connotations for people, which in fact provides a block to providing excellent pain and symptom management, and complete patient and family care.

According to the Canadian Hospice Palliative Care Association, hospice palliative care programs allow patients to gain more control over their lives, manage pain and symptoms more effectively, and provides support to family caregivers. [4]

Notes, thoughts, questions, and next chapter

Hospice palliative care aims to:
Treat all active issues.
Prevent new issues from occurring.
Promote opportunities for meaningful and valuable experiences, personal and spiritual growth, and self-actualization. [4]

You will find, at the end of each chapter, a place for your notes, thoughts, and questions. Please feel free to use your book as a companion on this, your journey, and take your book with your questions to your care providers to help start those difficult conversations. I highly recommend that you write down any ideas, questions, thoughts, and reflections that may be important to you. I encourage you to keep an open mind to the options that are available to help keep you comfortable and prepared for your journey.

In Chapter one, you have looked at some of the important topics that will be introduced in the following chapters. I hope that this chapter has shown you how the benefits of a palliative care approach can assist you in living and dying in comfort, and with dignity, in the setting of your own home. In the next chapter, you will learn the evolution of end-of-life care in the home; some strategies to begin to come to terms with your diagnosis and fears; how to re-frame hope; and how to begin the process of planning to stay home.

I thank you for choosing *The Book on Home Hospice: Living and Dying in Comfort with Dignity,* and I welcome you on this journey of discovery.

Now, let's get started!

Deborah Dooler, MD CCFP (PC) Palliative Care Physician

The best and most beautiful things in the world cannot be seen or even touched; they must be felt with the heart.
Helen Keller (1880-1968) deaf/blind author and activist

Notes

_____

_____

_____

_____

_____

_____

_____

_____

_____

_____

_____

_____

_____

_____

_____

_____

_____

_____

_____

_____

_____

_____

_____

_____

_____

_____

_____

Notes

Chapter 2
Home Hospice – Let's Take Your Journey Together

How people die remains in the memory
of those who live on.
Dame Cicely Saunders,
founder of the modern hospice movement

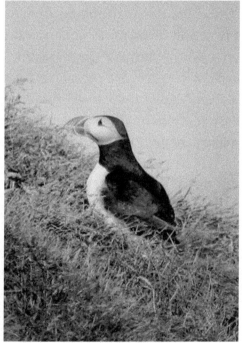

Photo.credit:Johnathon.Dooler2017

The Book of Home Hospice offers a comprehensive look at the philosophies and practical applications of providing care to those with a life-limiting illness, their caregivers, and support people as they journey together in their home. As the founder and medical director of the Niagara South Palliative Care Outreach Team, I have had a great deal of experience caring for palliative patients in the home. Working with the multidisciplinary team to assist people come to terms with their diagnosis, transition through the stages of grief, and maintain hope and ultimate acceptance and peace at end of life has been one of the most rewarding experiences of my life.

This chapter will give you an introduction to the history and evolution of end-of-life care in the home, from medieval times to modern day. It will help you to understand the stages of coming to terms with a terminal diagnosis, including denial, anger, bargaining, depression, and acceptance, as first described by Elizabeth Kubler-Ross, in 1969. It will introduce strategies to help you maintain and re-frame hope, and begin to make the necessary planning and preparations for staying at home.

Some helpful definitions:

Palliative care (also known as hospice palliative care, and end-of-life care) – The World Health Organization defines palliative care as "an approach that improves the quality of life of patients and their families facing the problems associated with life-threatening illness, through the prevention and relief of suffering, by means of early identification and impeccable assessment and treatment of pain and other problems, physical, psychosocial, and spiritual." [4]

Did You Know?
There are over 200 euphemisms for death in the English language. [12]
Some common euphemisms for death include:
•Fading quickly •Kick the bucket •Brown bread (cockney rhyming slang)
•Deceased •Departed •Demise •Expired •Gone to a better place
•Passed away •Passed on •Checked out •Bit the big one •Bitten the dust
•Popped their clogs •Pegged it •Taken to Jesus •Met his maker •Turned their toes up
•Cashed in their chips •Fallen off their perch •Croaked • Given-up the ghost
•Gone south •Shuffled off this mortal coil (from William Shakespeare's Hamlet)
•Pushing up daisies • Sleeping the big sleep •Checking out the grass from underneath
•Six feet under • the last breath •Paying a debt to nature

Hospice palliative care is an approach to care that aims to relieve suffering and improve the quality of living and dying, [4] in all settings, including the home, residential hospice, inpatient hospital palliative care unit, retirement home, and long-term care. It is appropriate for all ages and at all stages of disease progress. Grief and bereavement care for terminally ill people and their loved ones is an important part of hospice palliative care. [10]

Hospice may also refer to a free-standing building or unit in a hospital or long-term care facility providing end-of-life care, and acute palliative care units (PCU) providing care for the most difficult cases, from early diagnosis and not only those at end of life. [10]

End-of-life care – Palliative care provided in the last weeks and days of life, in any care setting.

Terminal illness – People may be diagnosed with a progressive, life-limiting or life-threatening illness; this may be cancer or non-cancer related.

Home hospice care – People with a terminal, life-limiting illness are provided care by a multidisciplinary team in their home.

Compassionate communities – In Canada, and around the world, the trend is towards seeing palliative care and dying as a public health issue. This compassionate community's model includes education and collaboration with community partners.

The evolution of end-of-life care in the home

It is impossible that anything so natural, so necessary, and so universal as death, should ever have been designed by providence as an evil to mankind.

Jonathan Swift (1667-1745) Irish-born English satirist

Throughout the centuries, the way we die has dramatically changed, with high infant and child mortality, death in childbirth, infectious diseases, and accidents being replaced by chronic diseases and cancer. In Canada, today, chronic diseases account for 70% of all deaths. [4]

In the Middle Ages, death was a community affair, while in the Victorian era, it became a part of family life and was predominantly home-based, with the dying loved one being cared for in the family bedroom, and laid out in the family parlor after death. In the 20th century, and with the advent of new medical technologies and hopes for new cures, most deaths were institutionalized. After World War II, attitudes towards death and dying changed significantly and, as a result, the majority of deaths have occurred away from home and families. [19]

Modern palliative care was developed from the hospice philosophy, founded by Dame Cicely Saunders, a British Physician, and aims to improve the quality of life for patients with life-threatening illness. [2] She started the St. Christopher's hospice in the United Kingdom, in the 1960s, to care for the dying. [14]

According to Canadian Hospice Palliative Care Association, the practice of hospice palliative care, in Canada, began in the 1970s and has evolved rapidly, adapting to keep pace with changes in people's experience of illness and dying. [4]

"For many years, hospice palliative care has focused on helping individuals and their families address these issues in the last few weeks of life. More recently, the palliative approach to care is being applied throughout the illness trajectory to help relieve suffering, improve the quality of life, engage people in their care, potentially prolong life, and strive for a comfortable death."[4] Addressing the need for palliative care in the home becomes more important than ever as national and international projections are showing a dramatic rise in the number of deaths due to increased life expectancy and large cohorts of *baby-boomers* reaching older age. [1] The capacity to care for the dying in institutionalized settings is under a great deal of strain. The current vision of providing hospice palliative care services in Ontario, Canada, and internationally, has again shifted to a vision for home-based care provided by a combination of professional and family caregivers. With this shift in philosophy, many communities are working towards ways of supporting the goal of a successful home hospice experience. The recent international compassionate community's initiative has been gaining strength over the past few years. The aim is to begin to normalize death and dying, and gain community

support systems to assist with the dying and bereaved. This could include school systems, and private and public businesses working collaboratively in partnership with the medical community to educate, raise awareness, and offer supports in the provision of palliative care, bringing full circle the idea of dying being a community event.

It is an exciting time for me to be working as a palliative care physician specialist in the field of home hospice. It is my hope that *The Book on Home Hospice* will be a helpful tool, for families and caregivers alike, to assist with the shifting trend towards communities building palliative care services from the ground up, and governments supporting palliative care services from the very top.

Much advocacy is needed to ensure that all those that wish to die at home have the access and opportunity that they so deserve in Canada and around the world.

*Free Resources at my website www.HomeHospice Book.com Please feel free to visit my site for directions on how access more information on how to advocate for palliative care services in your location.

Coming to terms with a terminal diagnosis

We must let go of the life we have planned,
so as to accept the one that is waiting for us.
Joseph Campbell

You are likely reading *The Book on Home Hospice* because you or a loved one has been given the news of a terminal illness. During this time, you may be feeling many different emotions about the diagnosis. The adjustment to the news and anticipatory grief (sadness and worry) of the expected losses is a normal yet challenging time. Each person's grief and adjustment is personal, and you may pass through many stages as you learn to cope and come to terms with your diagnosis.

- You may initially have feelings of shock, disbelief, and denial. You may be thinking, "No, it's not me; it cannot be true."

- You may wish to shield your family and friends, and continue to hope that the diagnosis is wrong.

- Denial can serve as a buffer to an unexpected shock, and is usually a temporary defense mechanism.

- Denial may be replaced with feelings of anger, rage, envy, and resentment. You might ask, "Why me?" "Why now?"

- You might be angry with those around you, including your family and doctors; you may be angry at God.

- The anger may be very difficult to cope with as it may be displaced and projected in many different ways, including guilt and blaming.

- Anger may lead to feelings of bargaining with God for more time. As this is a very private conversation, it can lead to feelings of isolation.

- When the time comes that you are unable to deny the illness any longer, you may have feelings of great loss, sadness, anxiety, and fear.

- Most people at the end of life are neither depressed nor angry, and they have had opportunity to mourn their impending loss and contemplate their coming death with a certain degree of inspection, and are able to die with peace and acceptance. [17] [18]

As a loved one and caregiver, this initial transition time can be frightening and challenging for you also. You may find you are struggling with your own emotions, fears, and anxieties, at the same time as you wish to support your loved one. The following are some ideas that may help you to understand and cope with this time of great emotional turmoil.

- Understand that the stages of grief are fluid and very personal. Stages may change back and forth from denial to anger, to bargaining, then depression, with final acceptance.

- At times, emotions may be directed towards family members, but these are likely projected fears and should not be taken personally.

- Be present to allow them to express their emotions, whether they be fears and anxieties, or feelings of joy and reminiscence.

- Remember the good times and the bad, using opportunities to connect them to their past.

- Do not avoid difficult conversations, and encourage any conflict resolution or unfinished business that may be outstanding.

- Respect privacy, and offer opportunities for conservation of dignity.

- Sometimes offering silence and companionship, without offering advice, can be helpful.

- Being a good listener is always supportive.

- Ask for help and support, if needed. You are not expected to have all the answers.

- You may not need to go through all stages with your loved one.

- Each person will progress at his or her own rate, in his or her own way.

You are braver than you believe, stronger than you seem, and smarter than you think.

AA Milne

When my youngest son, Johnathon, was 16 years old, he developed a fever with abdominal pain, and looked quite unwell. He had just returned from helping his sister, Amy, move into her apartment for her first year of nursing at Ryerson University. Our oldest son, Rick, had also just returned to Brock University that weekend, where he was studying accounting. My husband, John, and I brought him to the emergency department, suspecting appendicitis; within hours of the onset, he had his appendix removed in surgery. He was at home, recovering and doing quite well. At the time, I was working as a doctor in the hospital in which he had his surgery, and I knew his surgeon quite well, as his office was situated next door to mine. I remember being at work in the hospital and getting a page from the surgeon regarding a patient. This was common for me, as we often worked and looked after the same patient. The surgeon told me that the biopsy had come back positive for cancer, and it was a carcinoid tumor. I said, "Okay, thank you," and asked which patient he was talking about. He said, "Johnathon." I replied, "Johnathon who?" He replied, "Your son's biopsy came back as cancer." I continued with my disbelief, stating, "No, you must be mistaken; that cannot be so." He continued to tell me that during Johnathon's appendectomy surgery, he thought the appendix looked suspicious, and had sent it for a biopsy, which had confirmed that there was indeed a malignant tumor. Despite my years of medical education and experience, this news came as a complete shock to me. When I finally got off the telephone with the surgeon, I began to cry uncontrollably in the physician's lounge. I am so grateful that there were supportive people around me to ensure that I got home safely. Over the next short while, we continued to hope that the diagnosis was wrong, and we shielded our family, including Johnathon, from the news of the diagnosis. This was relatively short-lived as he needed to have further investigations and consultations. Our instinct was to protect and shield him as best as we could. I have very little recollection of the next few days and weeks while he was being tested and seeing consultants. Each family member came to terms with the situation in his or her own time and in their own way. In the end, it was determined that the tumor had been completely removed, and he has a done very well since then. I am certainly grateful for every day that I have to spend with my family. You will find photographs, taken by Johnathon while on a camping trip to Iceland, thorough out the book; I hope you enjoy them as much as I do.

---

*Hope is being able to see that there is light
despite all of the darkness.*
Desmond Tutu

Hope is the one thing that persists. Defense mechanisms and coping mechanisms help you to deal with the circumstances in a temporary manner. They may be replaced or exist side by side in a fluid flow from one state to another. There is always hope, and hope changes over time. When there is no longer hope for a cure, there can be hope for comfort, pain control, quality of life, closure, and a peaceful, relaxed, home experience.

Ask, if there was no hope for a cure, what else is possible to hope for, or worth looking forward to?

---

*Hope is the thing with feathers that perches in the soul...
And sings the tune without words, and never stops... At all.*
Emily Dickinson

The fear of death and dying

Hope is the only thing stronger than fear.
President Snow – The Hunger Games

Humans have been blessed with the virtue to be able to think and reason. This can be both a blessing and a curse. Coming to terms with your own mortality can cause what is known as death anxiety:

"a complex phenomenon that represents the blend of many different thought processes and emotions: the dread of death; the horror of physical or mental deterioration; the essential feeling of aloneness; the ultimate experience of separation, anxiety, and sadness about the eventual loss of self; and extremes of anger and despair about a situation over which we have no control." [14]

Fear can be caused by the awareness of potential suffering related to the progression of disease: [3] as an illness progresses, there may be a fear of becoming a burden on loved ones as the future becomes more uncertain, and physical changes may become apparent.

Some common fears:

Uncertainty of what comes beyond death
- Existential angst.
- Uncertainty of afterlife.
- Worry of going to heaven or hell.
- Worry of being nothing beyond.

Fears related to the dying process
- Fear of physical suffering.
- Embarrassment of losing control.
- Frustration with lack of mobility.
- Mortification of being totally dependent on others.

Fear of death as final separation from loved ones
- Feelings of aloneness, isolation, or disconnection.

Fear of shame and guilt
- Sense of guilt for one's body being deficient.
- Guilt for leaving children or parents to suffer.
- Survivor guilt (e.g., holocaust).
- Guilt from not having lived the fullest life.

Anguish and guilt
- Deep worry and concern about those left behind. [14]

Fear and worry about one's death is normal to our human experience. Sharing your feelings and concerns about death and dying, with your family or caregivers, is an important way to understand and overcome the fears that you may be experiencing. If things become overwhelming, seek help from your home care nurse for advice on counseling, or speak to your palliative or family physician. There are many options for counseling to overcome fear and grief.

You may be referred to a counselor, social worker, or chaplain. At times, there may be underlying childhood traumas, and therapies can be quite helpful to offer release at the end of life.

Spiritual support may be a welcome and necessary addition, if this is important to you. Prayer can be a comfort and can be helpful, if this is part of your journey. Some people may seek comfort in religion, while others are spiritual, and yet again others may look elsewhere. This may be a time for you to consider re-establishing ties with your religious community or spiritual beliefs.

It is important to be aware that your basic personality does not change throughout your life. How you deal with life is often how you will deal with death: coping mechanisms tend to be stable across time, and how you have dealt with trauma in the past is how you may anticipate dealing with future stress.

*Every man must do two things alone; he must do his own
believing and his own dying.*
Martin Luther King Jr.

Home sweet home – Choosing to be cared for in the comfort of your own home

Did You Know?
You are more likely to be killed by a champagne cork
than by a poisonous spider. [12]

Home is where the heart is. You may have heard this saying many times.   Just saying the word *home* may make you relax and smile. It is often said that a man is the king of his castle, or a woman is the queen of her castle, and who wouldn't want to stay in their own castle? In 2013, an international study of just over 100,000 people, from 33 countries, looking at preferences for place of care at the end of life or place of death, concluded that most people preferred a home death. [1]

Some of the reasons for this choice are:
1. The importance of being in a comfortable familiar place.
2. Being close to family and friends.
3. The ability to be close to pets.
4. Fear of hospitals.
5. Fear of change.

In my role as a palliative care physician, I have the privilege of caring for people as they journey with their life-limiting illness. I have witnessed the enormous rewards and benefits of staying home to die, and also some of the challenges and barriers people may face. The majority of people wish to stay at home as long as possible, sometimes with a plan for admittance to a residential hospice or another end-of-life institution as a back-up plan.

Your health care providers can help you and your caregivers to assess whether dying at home will be manageable. The following are some considerations from the College of Physicians and Surgeons of Canada [7]:

1. Your safety and the safety of those around you.
2. Your caregiver's ability to cope either physically or emotionally with the situation.
3. Whether the appropriate care can be provided (for example, round the clock coverage, if needed).
4. The availability of a home palliative care physician or family physician that makes home visits.
5. The availability of a community based palliative care team.
6. The viability of admittance to a residential hospice or other end-of-life bed, if needed.

Safety

When adapting your home to home hospice care, there are several things to consider. The layout of the home is extremely important to ensure safety and comfort for all involved. Your local home care coordinator can help you assess your home with the help of an occupational therapist or physiotherapist, and make suggestions for the most appropriate place for a bed, with access to bathroom facility or commode.

Infection Control

A most important consideration is infection control in the home environment, for the protection of everyone, including you and your family and healthcare providers.

Hand washing is the most effective way to prevent the spread of disease. Bacteria and viruses are carried on the hands, and can be removed by washing with warm soapy water. Hand washing should occur prior to any care provided, after any care provided, after going to the toilet, prior to eating, and after eating. Hand sanitizers should also be provided at points of care and at the bedside. Disposable gloves should be worn for any contact with body fluids, and disposed of appropriately, with dedicated garbage disposal units.

Needles and syringes should be discarded in appropriate containers.

Ensure all pets are up-to-date with vaccinations and are healthy.

Masks and gowns may be used if family or visitors have a bacterial or viral infection.

It is a nice idea to have a guest book at the front door for guests to sign as a remembrance of their visit.

It may be helpful to post a sign on the door and recommend that visitors do not visit if they have an infection, such as cold, flu, or pneumonia.

*Free Bonus Material at my website,
www.HomeHospiceBook.com.
Download a full-size, full-colour, print ready Door Sign.

Suggestions for things you can do to bring comfort and dignity

1. Offer a supportive, caring environment for your loved one to come to terms with a terminal diagnosis.
2. Provide the opportunity for maintaining privacy and dignity of your loved one.
3. Take care of your own needs, and ensure you are maintaining your own medical and dental appointments.
4. Keep important family routines, where possible; if necessary, let others go; ask for and accept help.
5. Avoid distancing yourself from your loved one, and ask for help when needed.
6. Ensure that you are able to get enough rest, sleeping while your loved one sleeps, if necessary.
7. Find ways to relieve your own stress, such as exercise, meditation, talking to friends or family, and seeking spiritual or religious support for yourself.

8. Ask for respite care from your healthcare provider if things become too much or overwhelming.
9. Safe storage of medications, especially narcotics and sedatives, in a lock box.
10. Store medications away from children, teens, and pets.
11. Do not throw medication packages in the recycling box to avoid alerting the neighbors.
12. Return all unused medications to the pharmacy.
13. Monitor for safe driving, cooking, etc. while taking narcotic or sedative medications.
14. Ensure safe disposal of all biohazard and medical supplies in appropriate containers.
15. Ensure your home has working smoke detectors, carbon monoxide detectors, and fire extinguishers. Check batteries monthly, and change batteries twice a year at daylight savings time; this is a good way to remember.
16. It is recommended to have a smoke detector in every bedroom, including the room you may be staying in for end of life, if it is not an official bedroom.
17. Monitor for placement of electric cords; remove all throw rugs to prevent trip hazard.
18. Ensure no smoking is allowed near oxygen.
19. Ensure no smoking is allowed in bed.

I don't know what to say – The etiquette of illness [56]

At times, it can be difficult to know just what to say to someone who has been diagnosed with a terminal illness. This can lead you to want to avoid contact with the ill person, as you may not know how to proceed.

- It's okay to say, "I don't know what to say."
- It's okay to ask, "Do you want to talk about it?"
- If you're wondering when would be a good time to call, the answer is, *anytime is a good time to call;* you can always leave a message saying, "Thinking of you."
- Sending cards and letters is a good way to offer your genuine thoughts.
- An email can be okay, if it's genuine and from the heart.
- If you fear saying the wrong thing, you can always just ask, "What is this like for you?"
- You can say, "I'm sorry you are facing this life challenge; do you want to talk about it?"
- If you don't know what to do, ask, "How can I help?"
- If the person is religious, offer your prayers.
- Sometimes just being there in silence, or listening, is okay.
- You may feel comfortable asking about the person's beliefs or thoughts and fears of dying.
- If you act from a place of love and compassion, you will find the words.

Special considerations for children and adolescents

 Even young children are capable of understanding the situation at the level of their development.

- Every attempt should be made to give opportunities for them to ask questions about the life-threatening illness.
- Take time to listen to their worries and fears.
- Answer questions honestly at a level that they are able to understand.
- Ensure that they understand they will not be left alone, and will be taken care of.
- Let them know that what's happening is not their fault.
- Let the school know what is happening.
- Keep visits short for small children.
- Allow them to help out in some way; for example, allowing artwork to decorate the space, and letting them help with small tasks.
- Always keep lines of communication open, especially with older children and teens.
- Offer to write letters or journal about their experiences and feelings.
- If family roles are changing, help children to learn to become proficient with unfamiliar tasks.

My notes, thoughts, questions, and next chapter

I highly recommend that you write down any ideas, questions, thoughts, and reflections that may be important to you. Please feel free to use your book as a companion on this, your journey, and take your book with your questions to your care providers to help start those difficult conversations.

In this chapter, you have taken a closer look at your emotions and feelings towards your diagnosis, and you have been given some strategies to help you cope. You are beginning to understand some steps necessary to start planning for your care in the home. In the very next chapter, you will find out how professional caregivers and loved ones can help bring comfort and dignity to you at home. Advance care planning will be discussed to help you to express your wishes in a way that ensures they will be followed.

It is my hope that *The Book on Home Hospice* will help you and your loved ones to gain the information and confidence you need to begin to gather your circle of care around you. You will find a dedicated group of professionals ready to go above and beyond to help you.

Laurie, a palliative community nurse, tells a story that shows the dedication and tenacity of the community visiting nurses.

"Early one morning, I was called to come early to see my 9 am patient, as he was in some distress. He was bedridden and lived in the middle of nowhere, in a place I like to call *Timbuktu*. So, I headed out to see him and arrived at his property, to find all the doors to be locked. I called the home phone and found the line was dead—probably left off the hook. I knocked on the door and called out, but since he was bedridden, and his wife was deaf, I got no response. Things just didn't seem right to me. I didn't give up. I thought I would try the backyard, but the gate was locked. As I peeked around into the back, I could see his bedroom window was open slightly, and I heard him struggling to breathe. You should know I am a large woman, and I have had a hip replacement, so I don't usually attempt any acrobatics. However, time was of the essence, so I climbed over a three-foot fence into the yard, and yelled, "I'm coming, Ralph!" Once in the yard, I could see the window, but it was four feet off the ground. I could hear his wheezing getting worse. I shouted, "Don't worry, Ralph; I will get to you!" Frantically looking for something to climb on, I found a wheelbarrow and tipped it upside down. I scrambled onto the barrow and tossed my bag in through the open window. I heaved myself through the window and landed on his hospital bed with a thud. Once in the room, I gave him his Ventolin treatment and took my own Ventolin puffer. And when we both had settled down, Ralph asked, "Did you leave the wheelbarrow in place?" I answered, "Yes, why?" He said, "I want you to do the same thing tomorrow morning, so I can video tape it!" We laughed so hard, we could barely breathe. Well, he didn't videotape my acrobatics, but we did set up a video camera in his yard, so he could watch his over 50 Rhododendron plants grow in the garden.

Now, that is what I call dedication and commitment.

Notes

_____

_____

_____

_____

_____

_____

_____

_____

_____

_____

_____

_____

_____

_____

_____

_____

_____

_____

_____

_____

Chapter 3
Your Circle of Care

There are only four kinds of people in this world: those who have been caregivers; those who are currently caregivers; those who will be caregivers; those who will need caregivers.
Rosalynn Carter,
former first lady of the United States of America

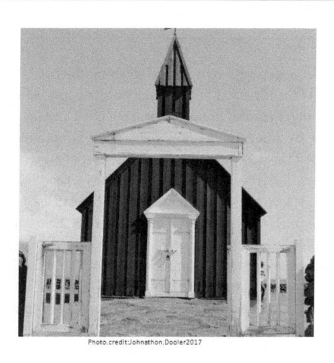

Photo.credit:Johnathon.Dooler2017

Home hospice care brings together a multi-service, multidisciplinary team of professionals, volunteers, family, and loved ones, in the circle of care around you. In this chapter of *The Book on Home Hospice,* you will learn about the members of the team and their roles. You will explore your own role and responsibilities as a team member, and learn about the importance of advance care planning.

You are the navigator of your own health care.
Sue Battersby-Campbell,
Palliative Community Outreach Nurse Practitioner

Sue is an outreach nurse practitioner on the palliative care team, and she loves her home hospice visiting role. She states, "People don't ask me to save their life; I can't anyway. People want to be home, and they want their symptoms to be managed. I can do that, and it is the best part of my work." Sue is outgoing and gregarious, and a force to be reckoned with. She declares, "I love humor, I love to banter, and I can learn exactly how a person is feeling by asking questions. I ask them what they did yesterday, how their garden is doing, and what is on the agenda for the weekend. I find people do not want to be treated with kid gloves, and humor can often be overlooked by healthcare professionals." She encourages people to put the living back into life by getting dressed and groomed every day, if possible. Sue is a big advocate for taking responsibility for your own health and life, maintaining that you are the navigator of your own health care, and you can't depend on everyone else. "You should know about you." She encourages people to "get a journal, keep a list, write it down, and take it with you." "Not talking about things does not make them any less real," she maintains. "There is great suffering in silence."

Some helpful definitions:

Caregiver – A caregiver is an individual who provides ongoing care and assistance, without pay, for family members and friends in need of support due to physical, cognitive, or mental health conditions. [4]

Caregiver Burnout – The word *burnout* describes the exhaustion of physical or emotional strength.

Circle of Care – It is a term commonly used to describe the ability of certain health information custodians to assume an individual's implied consent to collect, use, or disclose personal health information for the purpose of providing health care, in circumstances defined in PHIPA. [22]

The Personal Health Information Protection Act – Also known as PHIPA. [22]

The philosophy of home hospice care

The topic of end of life is on people's minds. Three-quarters of Canadians (74%) report having thought about end of life, with the vast majority of Canadians believing hospice palliative care has a positive impact. [4] According to the Canadian Hospice Palliative Associations report, *Model to Guide Hospice Palliative Care 2013,* hospice palliative care is most effectively delivered by an inter-professional team of healthcare providers who form therapeutic relationships with the person and family. [4] Family and informal caregivers, providing hospice palliative care at home, are undertaking a wider range of tasks in an environment where they typically have less support from professional caregivers. Tasks assigned to family and informal caregivers may include psychological, social, and spiritual care; personal care; medical care, including administration of medications and injections; homemaking services; and advocacy and care-coordination. The average number of hours per week that Canadians spend caring for a dying family member is 54.4 hours. Based on a study in Ontario, palliative care clients were cared for primarily by their spouses or partners (57%), or their children or children-in-law (29%). Over one-quarter (28%) of caregivers, or 2.2 million individuals, could be considered sandwiched between caregiving and raising children. Most of them were women between the ages 35 and 44, helping their parents or parents-in-law, while also having at least one child under 18 living at home. [4]

The philosophy of hospice palliative care is driven by the following four values:

1. **Autonomy.** You have the right to make your own decisions.
2. **Self-Actualization.** Dying is part of living and may be an opportunity for you to grow.
3. **Dignity.** You have the right to be treated with dignity and integrity.
4. **Community.** A unified response to suffering strengthens communities. [4]

Canadian Hospice Palliative Care Association Model

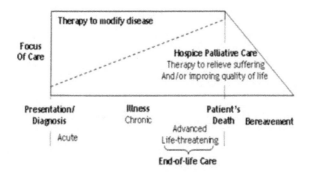

Types of Care – Even though the plan includes care and death at home, there may be times where your needs may be met in a different setting. [14]

Types of care	Settings of care
1. **Acute care**: For issues that require time-limited attention.	- Acute care hospitals, including emergency rooms, intensive care units, medical, surgical, obstetric, pediatric, geriatric, and rehabilitation
2. **Chronic care**: Issues that require continuous support and/or skilled nursing care.	- Individual homes - Complex continuing care - Palliative care unit in hospital or long-term care- Free-standing residential hospice- Long-term homes
3. **Respite care**: When caregivers become fatigued and require a break or a vacation.	- Day programs - Individual homes- Long-term homes
4. **End-of-life care**: When issues and the need for care can arise considerably, and particularly in the last days of life.	- All settings
5. **Bereavement care**: For those who survived the person's death.	- All settings

Professional Caregivers – Bringing comfort and dignity to you at home

---

Alone we can do so little; together we can do so much.

Helen Keller (1880-1968) deaf/blind author and activist

In my role as a visiting palliative care physician on a busy outreach community palliative care team, it is my privilege to work with an exceptional group of home care professionals, including nurse practitioners, clinical navigators, administrative assistants, psychosocial bereavement clinicians, palliative nurses, personal support workers, care coordinators, dieticians, hospice inpatient and day hospice staff, chefs, and volunteers. Everyone's goal is the same: to make you the centre of the circle of care, and bring a special quality and expertise to the team.

Their dedication and commitment to providing compassionate care at home is evident. Jocelyn is a palliative home care nurse with many years of community experience. I interviewed Jocelyn and asked her what she felt was the most rewarding thing about her work. She stated, "People can focus on the quality of life and not so much on the time remaining, making the most of what time they have left, and making it better." She pronounced, "Let's make the journey there more fulfilling for them. The sooner we can get working on things, the more peaceful the ending."

She maintains that, "Home palliative care is by far the most fulfilling nursing I have ever done. I'm able to see people through to the most vulnerable end. To be allowed into their home and treat them is a privilege. A person in their home is not just a patient; you are able to get to know them as an individual: what they do for a living; what their likes and dislikes are; what is important to them; and their family, pets, and hobbies. People are more comfortable if they can stay in their natural habitat. In the hospital, it was less personal. In the home, they are mother, grandmother, and aunt, and have lived a life. They can be themselves."

She tells them, "Don't clean the house, and don't get out of your pajamas. We come to you as you are; we become part of the family." She finds most rewarding the ability to help people to find peace, comfort, and dignity through their journey, while making them the centre of the experience.

Palliative care team member roles [14]

Case manager/care coordinator – The role of the case manager includes assessment, information and linking, service planning, and evaluation of home care services.

Clergy/spiritual/pastoral care – The rule of the clergy and pastoral care is to assess the spiritual needs, and offer support for grief and bereavement.

Clinical navigator and administrative support staff – The role of the clinical navigator and administrative support staff is to assist the care team to organize and plan visits and meetings.

Hospice palliative care volunteers – The role of the volunteer is to provide practical assistance with support, listening, and advocacy.

Nurse – The role of the registered nurse/registered practical nurse is to a function within the scope of practice, including assessment, therapeutic encounters, collaborating with team members, education, and symptom control.

Nurse practitioner – The role of the nurse practitioner is to function within the scope of practice, including assessment, therapeutic encounters, ordering diagnostic tests, prescribing some medications, and educating and mentoring other team members.

Occupational therapist – The role of the occupational therapist is to provide goals for daily activity and self-care productivity and leisure, to maintain quality of life and safety.

Personal support worker and health care aide – The role of the personal support worker or health care aide is to assist with activities of daily living, including personal care, nutrition, light housekeeping, laundry, and respite.

Pharmacist – The role of the pharmacist is to prepare, dispense, and distribute medications, and complete medication assessments.

Family physician – The role of the family physician is to assess the medical needs of the person and family, to provide ongoing medical care support and guidance, and to link to specialty physicians and teams, such as radiation, oncology, etc.

Palliative care physician –The role of the palliative care physician is to act as a medical advisor consultant to the team liaison between medical staff and palliative care team, and to provide medical, emotional, social, and spiritual support, including ordering diagnostic tests and ordering medications.

Physician assistants – This is a new role being introduced into Ontario and elsewhere to help support the physicians.

Physiotherapist – The role of physiotherapist is to assess and improve mobility and consequences of a lack of mobility.

Recreational therapist – The role of the recreational therapist is to provide an activities program and social visits.

Registered dietitian – The role of the registered dietitian is to assess nutrition status and develop an individual nutrition care plan.

Respiratory therapist – The role of the respiratory therapist is to assist in developing a plan to address respiratory issues.

Social worker – The role of the social worker is to assess psychosocial needs, and develop a care plan.

Speech language – The role of the speech language pathologist is to assess for communication and swallowing issues.

Susan is a clinical navigator on the palliative care team. She asserts, "I have the satisfaction of knowing that I am working with wonderful people who make a large difference in the lives of other people." Susan is the team's miracle maker; she goes above and beyond to advocate for people, and she works hard to make each person's experience meaningful to them. She states, "I put myself in their situation and think of what I would want someone to do for me. I am always thinking of ways to make someone feel better; I am just being human." She has worked with many community partners to have special things arranged and donated. In one such example, she arranged for a family portrait for a family with a dying two-year-old daughter. The picture is a treasured memory that they will have forever. She has arranged for camping holidays, hotel stays with limo rides to Niagara Falls, and a resort holiday at Sherkston Resort. She maintains, "Don't be afraid to ask your questions. If there is something you need or want, you never know; you may be able to get these things."

Loved ones as caregivers

The simple Act of caring is heroic.
Edward Albert

Completing the circle of care around their terminally ill loved ones are family, friends, and neighbors as caregivers. Kim is a palliative care nurse with over 30 years of home care experience. Kim affirms, "My motto is that I can't change where you're going, only how you get there. I can help with comfort, number 1, coping, number 2, and passing nicely with dignity, number 3. In the home setting, you get to know people and their families, and you are able to respect their limits and ask them at the beginning of their journey what it is that they want."

Every house is personalized to the individual and, in every interaction, family are involved in the circle of care. You have the time to be able to explain and show things to people. She regrets that sometimes if she gets called in too late, and a person wants to die at home, it is difficult to make the necessary arrangements. This is frustrating for all involved. She admits it is easier having access to the palliative care team, physician, nurse practitioner, and counsellors, as most family practitioners do not do home visits or have after hours palliative call coverage, and they are uncomfortable prescribing the palliative medications needed to provide comfort in the home. This can lead to unresolved symptoms, emergency department visits, or hospital admission. Adequate access to multidisciplinary palliative care teams across the country remains an issue.

I had the great honor of meeting and caring for Kim's mother, Dorothy, at the end of her life, in her daughter's home. Kim's mother, just like Kim, was a feisty, redhead, fireball. It was wonderful to see both mother and daughter in the home with their tiny little red-headed Yorkie-Poo named Pearl.

With the team set in place, Kim's mother passed quickly, quietly, peacefully, and with dignity in her daughter's home. I was able to respect and treat Kim as a daughter, and not as a nurse. Kim declares, "It was a beautiful death, if you can say death is beautiful."

Dorothy had the very common concern about being a burden to her family. Kim ensured her that was not the case, stating, "You've taken care of me my whole life; it is my time to take care of you. I'm giving you this gift."

She expresses, "It reminded me of the book, *I Love You Forever,* written by Robert Munsch, where the child sits and rocks mother at the end. It was an experience that none of us will forget or regret."

Advanced Care Planning – Expressing your wishes

The best preparation for tomorrow is doing your best today.
H. Jackson Brown Jr.

The Canadian Medical Association recommends that all Canadians should have an advanced care plan [6], also known as advanced directive, personal directive, or living will. This is to ensure that the health care team follow your wishes should you become unable to express them. An advanced care plan is a way of expressing your wishes for your health plan, should you become unable to do so. This can be done verbally by telling your proxy decision maker your wishes, or it can be written. In Canada, it is the law that the capable patient always decides. [5] Planning for end of life can ensure that the care provided to you aligns with your wishes, values, and beliefs. [7]

You are determined to be capable for making your own treatment decisions if you are able to understand the proposed treatment, and you can appreciate the consequences of accepting or refusing the treatment.

Some helpful definitions:

Advanced Care Plan – A way to express your health care wishes should you be unable to do so (also known as advanced directive, personal directive, or living will).

Cardiopulmonary resuscitation CPR – A potentially lifesaving intervention that is provided with the intention of reversing or interrupting a potentially fatal event (e.g., cardiac or respiratory arrest). CPR is often understood to include chest compressions, artificial ventilation, and defibrillation. [7]

Do Not Resuscitate (DNR) – (also known as *Allow Natural Death)* You may express a wish to not be resuscitated. Your physician or nurse are advised to order and complete the Ministry of Health and Long-Term Care *Do Not Resuscitate Confirmation Form.* This will direct the emergency services that no heroic measures are to be performed. [7] You can change your mind at any time.

Life-sustaining treatment – Any medical procedure or intervention that utilizes mechanical or other artificial means to sustain, restore, or supplant a vital function essential to the life of the patient (e.g., mechanical ventilation, medically assisted nutrition, and hydration, etc.). [7]

Potentially life-saving treatment – Treatment that is provided with the intention of reversing or interrupting a potentially fatal event (e.g., cardiopulmonary resuscitation, defibrillation, artificial respirations). [7]

Power of attorney for personal care – The substitute decision maker that you choose to make health care decisions for you, with a premade document, while you are capable to do so.

Power of attorney for finance – The person that you choose to make financial decisions for you, with a premade document, while you are capable to do so.

Substitute decision maker – The person who is legally able to decide about treatment options for you if you are unable to. In the absence of a power of attorney for personal care, each province has a hierarchy for selecting a legal substitute decision maker.

Free Bonus Material

To view the hierarchy outlined in the Ontario Consent to Treatment Act (1996), go to my website at www.HomeHospice Book.com.

Suggestions for things you can do to bring comfort and dignity

1. **Things to consider before taking on the commitment of primary caregiver:**
   How will I juggle my work and my children in the day-to-day care of someone I love so much?
   Can I take a leave of absence from work?
   Is it a role I am suited to?
   Will I have the physical and emotional strength, or the practical support that I will need?
   Is it desirable or physically possible for me to care for a dying person in my home? [26]

2. **You can't pour from an empty cup; take care of yourself first.**

3. **Caregiver Burnout**
   Signs and symptoms of caregiver burnout are similar to those for depression:
   Withdrawal from family and friends.
   Loss of interest in activities.
   Feeling down and irritable.
   Change in appetite, weight loss, or weight gain.
   Altered sleep patterns.
   Getting sick more often.
   Emotional and physical exhaustion.

It's not selfish to love yourself, take care of yourself,
and to make your happiness a priority.
It's a necessity.

Steps to avoid burnout

- Talk to someone you trust, such as a friend, a co-worker, your family physician, or home hospice team.
- Set realistic goals for yourself; you may not be able to do everything on your own. It is okay to ask for help.
- Take care of yourself, and set aside time for your own needs to ensure that you maintain your own physical health and fitness. Ensure you continue with your own medical and

dental appointments. You need to be healthy in order to take care of your loved one.

When to call for help:

- The urge to run and hide from responsibility becomes strong.
- Your activity is scattered and frantic.
- There is a major change in your sleeping patterns or eating habits.
- You are often irritable or easily angered.
- You cannot concentrate and are forgetting important details.
- You use alcohol, drugs, or tobacco more than before.
- You lose more than 10 lbs, or sleep less than 3 hours, or cannot read more than a few sentences without losing concentration..

4. **Complete your advanced care directive**

   Ensure your family are aware of your wishes.
   Complete your will, and living will, including plans for your digital legacy.
   Complete your power of attorney for healthcare and finance.

*Free Resources

To access the resource, "Speak Up, Canadian Virtual Hospice and Advance Care Planning Resource for Patients," go to my website at www.HomeHospiceBook.com.

Did you know?
You are more likely to die from a falling coconut than from a shark attack

My notes, thoughts, questions, and next chapter

I highly recommend that you write down any ideas, questions, thoughts, and reflections that may be important to you. Please feel free to use your book as a companion on this, your journey, and take your book with questions to your care providers to help start those difficult conversations.

Now you have been introduced to the people in your circle of care, and you have learned the importance of completing your advanced care plan. The next chapter will begin to introduce strategies you and your loved ones can use to recognize, monitor, and relieve suffering from physical symptoms, and ensure that you are in comfort.

Notes

Chapter 4
Relief of Common Symptoms of the Body

Cure sometimes, treat often, comfort always.
Hippocrates

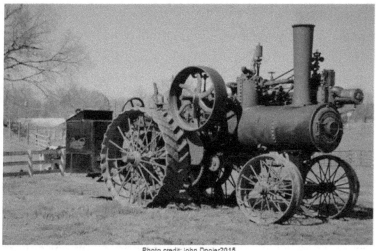

Photo.credit:John.Dooler2015

How to recognize and relieve physical suffering

The palliative care approach has the aim to achieve comfort by relieving suffering and distress, and to improve the quality of living and dying for those with a life-limiting illness. In this chapter of *The Book on Home Hospice,* you will learn the basic approach to recognize, monitor, and aim to relieve the physical suffering due to pain, breathing issues, general decline in energy and appetite, gastrointestinal issues, skin wounds and, lastly, urinary and sexual concerns.

Over 3 in 10 Canadians (32%) personally suffer from a chronic illness, while 4 in 10 (39%) have a sufferer in their immediate family. When taken together, 6 in 10 Canadians are impacted by chronic illness. [4] As chronic conditions are increasingly leading causes of death, most people should expect a period of terminal illness to precede death [1], during which time the body can experience symptoms of distress.

Identifying distress in the person with severe communication difficulty can be challenging; however, even comatose people can show signs or behaviors of distress. Partners and relatives can provide valuable information, and especially in children, their perspective is essential. This includes adults or children with severe learning disability, people with dementia, severe dysphasia (stroke, cerebral tumor), severe depression or psychosis, or in a comatose or semi-comatose state. [10]

What are the behaviors and signs of distress?

Verbal: This may be simple statements, e.g. "I'm not right," or crying, screaming, sighing, moaning, or grunting.

Facial: These may be simple expressions (grimacing, clenched teeth, shut eyes, wide open eyes, frowning, biting lower lip) or more complex.

Adaptive: Rubbing or holding an area, keeping an area still, breath-holding, hyper-sensitivity to stimuli, approaching staff, avoiding stimulation, reduced or absent function (reduced movement, lying, or sitting).

Distractive: Rocking (or other rhythmic movements), pacing, biting their hand or lip, gesturing, clenched fists.

Postural: Increased muscle tension, altered posture, flinching, head in hands, or limping.

Autonomic: This may be either sympathetic (the flight or fright response with increased pulse rate, increased blood pressure, wide pupils, pallor [pale skin], and sweating) or a parasympathetic in response to nausea or visceral (abdominal organ) pain with decreased blood pressure and pulse rate.

Pain

Pain is the subjective feeling of physical suffering or discomfort in the body, and may be described as tender, aching, throbbing, stinging, twinging, burning, stabbing, or dull, and may be either constant or intermittent.

People often have multiple problems as the cause for their pain. In advanced cancer, for example, 85% of people have more than one site of pain, and 40% have 4 or more pains. Up to 85% of people with advanced cancer will experience pain [10], and up to 60% of people with AIDS will experience neuropathic (nerve) pain. [10]

Diagnosing and treating pain is the role of the palliative care team or the family physician, oncology team or specialist team. The first point of contact in the home is most likely the home care nurse. The specially trained nurse will assess the nature, severity, and character of the pain.

If medications have been prescribed, they should be administered and taken as directed.

The nurse will contact the appropriate physician for changes in orders and to ask for a further assessment if needed.

When to call for help:
- New onset of severe pain not relieved with regular or breakthrough medication.
- New pain in the spine or limbs that may be an indication of a fracture in the bone.
- Worsening of pain that had previously being maintained.

Most adults and older children can clearly describe pain and its nature. It is important to ask how the pain has affected them. The basic rule is that "pain is what the person says hurts."

Severe or overwhelming pain – Pain of this severity needs urgent treatment.

Breakthrough pain – A brief, worsening of pain can *break through* the analgesia, resulting in distress.

Causes of breakthrough pain are related to movement or a procedure, inadequate regular analgesia, an unpredictable worsening of the pain (e.g. pathological fracture episodic pain caused by a pain less responsive to the current analgesia), or reluctance of the patience to take analgesia because of misunderstanding adverse effects, or the fear of adverse effects. [27]

The choice of pain medication that your physician or nurse practitioner chooses may depend on:

- The cause of the pain.
- The route of administration.
- Your preference for preparation.
- Coexisting conditions such as kidney and liver impairment.
- Adverse effects, medical precautions, and contradictions.
- The need for combination analgesia.

Side effects of pain medications to monitor for:

Drowsiness – Medication can have an effect on the nervous system and cause a person to become more sleepy or drowsy.

Respiratory depression – Some medications can slow the breathing down; this should be reported immediately if suspected. At the end of life, breathing does become irregular and slow, as a part of the normal disease progression.

Nausea and vomiting – When starting a new medication, this can be a problem, and may disappear in a few days, or your physician may recommend an anti-nausea medication, to be taken prior to the dose.

Constipation – Opioids can slow down the gut and cause constipation; you should routinely take a bowel stimulant and stool softener to help alleviate this.

Confusion – There may be mild confusion or possibly hallucination as a side effect of medications. This should be reported and may need to be treated.

Myoclonus – This is twitching or spasm of the muscles.

Addiction or physical dependence – Physical dependence is the body's response to the medication, while addiction is a psychological dependence, or the need to feel high from medication. If you have concerns regarding this, please speak to your medical practitioner.

Tolerance – The body may need a higher dose of medication over time as it adjusts.

For up-to-date information on opioid safety, please go to the Canadian virtual hospice website, an excellent evidence-based resource online. [36]

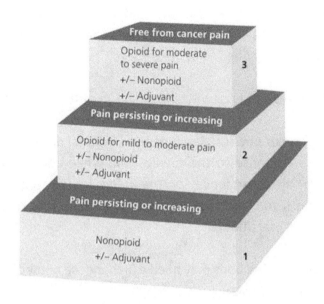

(WHO) World Health Organization
Ladder for pain control

Your physician may use the World Health Organization ladder for pain control to choose the best option for you, to ease your suffering and maintain your comfort.

Medicinal marijuana cannabis

Medicinal marijuana is legal in Canada and other States and jurisdictions around the world. Individuals with medical needs may have authorization from their healthcare provider to access cannabis. [37] It is formulated into a dried leaf product for smoking, vaping, or baking into food and oil. Your healthcare provider may offer a referral to a cannabis specialized clinic to determine your specific needs.

Medical marijuana can be helpful with symptoms such as pain, nausea, and decreased appetite.

Cannabinoids are the active chemical ingredients produced by the cannabis plant. More than 100 different cannabinoids have been identified, but research has focused on only two of them so far: delta-9-tetrahydrocannabinol (THC), and cannabidiol (CBD). [38] After assessment, your medical professional will determine the best combination of THC and CBD for your specific symptoms. In Canada, on July 1st, 2018, marijuana will be legal for sale for recreational use, in addition to medicinal use. It is currently available for recreational use in some states and countries around the world.

Caution
As police and health officials are warning that marijuana and other drugs could be laced with fentanyl, carfentanil, or other illicit drugs, it is extremely important to use only pure marijuana from a known safe source.

Opioid overdose crisis

The opioid overdose crisis refers to a recent increase in opioid deaths due to overdose in Canada and throughout the world. The issue stems from the illegal use of fentanyl or carfentanil, and other opioids, which are being used for non-medical purposes. Fentanyl is a man-made opioid that is 50 to 100 times more potent than morphine. Carfentanil is chemically similar to fentanyl but 10,000 times more potent than morphine. Carfentanil has no use in humans due to its extreme toxicity, its primary purpose being to tranquilize large animals such as elephants. Fentanyl and carfentanil are being added to illicit drugs such as oxycodone and heroin. Police and health officials are warning that marijuana and other drugs could be laced with fentanyl, carfentanil, or other illicit drugs. Governments around the world are acknowledging and attempting to put policies in place to protect against opioid deaths. [36]

Diversion, misuse, and abuse

Diversion, misuse, and abuse are potential problems.

Drug diversion – A medical and legal concept involving the transfer of any legally prescribed controlled substance from the individual for whom it was prescribed to another person for any illicit use.

Drug misuse – Refers to the illegal or illicit drug taking or alcohol consumption that leads a person to experience social, psychological, physical, or legal problems related to intoxication or regular excessive consumption and/or dependence.

Drug abuse – The compulsive, excessive, and self-damaging use of habit forming drugs or substances, leading to addiction.

Caution
Contact your health care providers or the police if you have concerns regarding the illegal use of your medications.

Breathing

Patrick is one of my regular palliative care clients that I follow routinely at home. He has been diagnosed with lung cancer and end-stage Chronic Obstructive Pulmonary Disease (COPD).He struggles with breathlessness. I asked him about his experience with the palliative care team program and how it has impacted his life. He stated:

"When I first got home from the hospital, I thought I would need to go into a nursing home. I was in pretty rough shape. That's when I met Colleen, my palliative home care nurse. She said, "I can get you help and keep you here at home." Getting help is half the battle to staying at home. She referred me to the palliative care team, and I started getting home visits from Dr. Dooler, and Sue, the nurse practitioner. Sue gave me some really good ideas to help with my breathing, which I still use to this day. She helped me gain the confidence to be able to stay home safely and manage my symptoms.

Since being followed closely by Dr. Dooler and the team, I have had no emergency department visits or hospital admissions in the last 2 years. I contribute it to the close monitoring of my symptoms, and stand-by medication orders at my pharmacy for prednisone and an antibiotic to start as soon as my nurse notices symptoms.

I have only been off my property twice in the last 2 years, which I think helps me to avoid getting infections, but I don't mind. My circle of life is small but manageable, and not at all depressing. I have lived a full life and I am able to enjoy watching my granddaughter grow up. I am very comfortable with my lifestyle right now. And I don't miss anything, especially the frequent emergency department visits and hospital admissions. Some people think I might be a recluse or loner, but I don't see it that way. I live with my son and granddaughter, and I have family visit daily to bring me food. The caregivers that have come into my life have been a blessing. I have happy people come into my home to help me every day and brighten my life: the personal support workers really enhance my lifestyle by treating me with respect and dignity."

Colleen maintains, "I really enjoy my visits with Patrick; we have fun and talk about life, and I have become part of the family. At first, Patrick was reluctant to try some of the suggestions, such as a small dose of morphine for his breathing, but as I gained his trust, he was willing to give it a try."

Patrick affirms, "I was reluctant to accept any help at first, but Colleen's attention to detail and expert assessments helped me to gain her trust. I started the morphine ordered by Dr. Dooler, and it has helped me breathe much better; I'm still ticking. Being in my own home is such a comfort; I would highly recommend the palliative care team program to anyone who wants to stay out of the hospital. I am also very grateful to the support counsellor, Clare, for helping my family cope with my illness, as it has impacted all of us. I have nothing but gratitude for the whole program."

Colleen is a palliative care community nurse with many years' experience, working to help people live and die in comfort with dignity and to stay in their own homes. She asserts that it is most satisfying to see Patrick in good spirits despite his ongoing struggles with breathing. To know that she has been able to improve his quality of life, and offer some happiness to him on her visits, makes it all worthwhile.

Shortness of breath, also called dyspnea, is the subjective feeling of suffering caused by not being able to get enough air or oxygen, and can often be described as intense tightening in the chest, air hunger, or the feeling of suffocation. Breathlessness is what you say it is, and is often frightening. Managing and relieving shortness of breath is essential to maintaining your comfort.

Breathlessness is the most common breathing problem, being present in 94% of chronic lung disease patients, 83% of heart failure patients, and up to 70% of cancer patients, but it is also common in dementia, multiple sclerosis, and AIDS.

Treatment of breathlessness

Mild facial cooling reduces breathlessness and discomfort. Blow a fan across the face or open a window.

Sitting upright increases peak ventilation and reduces airway obstruction.

Pursed lip breathing (PLB) is a breathing technique that consists of exhaling through tightly pressed lips (pursed lips), and inhaling through the nose with the mouth closed.

*Free Bonus Material at my website, www.HomeHospice Book.com.

When to call for help:
- You have new onset of symptoms suddenly, and not part of the end-of-life changes.
- You have chest pain.
- You have thick yellow, green, or bloody mucus.
- You cannot get a proper breath for more than 3 minutes.
- Skin is pale, blue, cool, and clammy.
- You have a fever..

Some helpful definitions:

Excess secretions – Thick airway secretions need to be loosened. Nebulized saline is often helpful.

Pleural effusions – Excess fluid accumulates in the pleural cavity (the space that surrounds the lungs). Drainage of the lung, called thoracentesis, may be considered if you are distressed.

Radiotherapy and chemotherapy – These can help in responsive lung tumors.

Respiratory infections – Most cases, the disease will progress, regardless of antibiotics.

Hiccups – Gastric stasis can cause hiccups and should be treated.

Cough – No one preparation has been shown to be consistently effective.

Persistent Breathlessness – Drugs used to treat breathlessness – apart from bronchodilators and antibiotics, other drugs have a limited role in breathlessness.

Opioids – Can reduce the demand for ventilation without significant respiratory depression, in cancer, end-stage heart failure, and chronic obstructive pulmonary disease (COPD). There is no evidence that opioids decrease survival, even in high doses.

Sedation – This is not usually the aim when managing breathlessness, but occasionally severe breathlessness that develops suddenly at the end of life (e.g. pulmonary embolus) will need sedation. Midazolam is usually preferred because its short half-life allows doses to be adjusted.

Non-invasive ventilation NIV – Ventilation can significantly improve the quality of life for patients with chronic hypercapnic respiratory failure due to progressive neuromuscular disease (e.g. motor neuron disease/ALS, Duchenne muscular dystrophy) or chronic obstructive pulmonary disease.

Breathlessness at the end of life – Causes distress and fear, sometimes with gasping respiration. This uncontrolled breathlessness can cause intense distress in people, partners, and relatives. Lorazepam or midazolam can be helpful for patients.

Loose airway secretions at the end of life – Can be a problem in up to 92% of patients in the last hours, or occasionally days, of a patient's life. Most comatose patients seem unaware of its presence, but it is distressing for loved ones to watch (also called *death rattle)*.

Fatigue, drowsiness, lethargy, and weakness

In a 2013 study, "Symptoms, ability, and the nature of suffering in terminal cancer patients dying at home: A prospective study," researchers reported that weakness was the most prevalent unbearable symptom in an end-of-life primary care cancer population. [3]

Fatigue is defined as extreme tiredness, and can cause a combination of mental and physical suffering. It is the most common symptom in advanced disease, and is reported in up to 80% of people. Drowsiness, tiredness, lethargy, fatigue, and weakness have different meanings for different people.

Reversible causes may be considered, but tiredness, fatigue, drowsiness, lethargy, and weakness are also a part of the natural dying process. If the reduced alertness is sudden, your physician or nurse may check for hypoxia (low blood oxygen level), hypercapnia (high carbon dioxide level), bleeding, cardiac arrhythmia (irregular heart rhythm), respiratory depression (slow breathing), and recently administered drugs.

Treating the cause

Nutrition – This is important in the earlier stages of any disease. In the later stages of the disease progression, the body will not need as much food or nutrition.

Modifying activities that cause fatigue – Activities are changed by using rest periods between activities, and re-timing activities to a time of day when energy is highest.

Medications – There is little evidence that drugs have any long-term benefit. However, corticosteroids remain an option for short-term use, and dexamethasone, 2–4 mg, can give a short-term improvement for up to four weeks. Psychostimulants are occasionally used: examples are methylphenidate and modafinil.

Swelling, edema, and lymphedema

Edema is a condition characterized by an excess of watery fluid collecting in the cavities or tissues of the body. Lymphedema is a specific term given to edema caused by impairment of lymph drainage. Treatment is centered on skin care and limb positioning, together with support, exercise, massage, and containment bandaging or hosiery.

The medical team's assessment of the edema should include:

- Speed of onset and distribution.
- Appearance of the skin (color, temperature, integrity, consistency).
- Associated symptoms (pain, sensory changes, restlessness).

When to call for help:
Features suggesting urgent investigation
These include the sudden onset of edema, pain (edema is not usually painful), new distended veins, skin color changes, and breathlessness.

Causes of swelling include:

Acute vena cava obstruction – Obstruction of the superior vena cava (a short, wide vessel carrying circulating blood into the heart from the body). Sudden onset (hours to days), bilateral (both sides) limb edema (with or without midline edema of head or genitals), soft pitting edema, and a dusky, purplish hue are features of superior vena cava obstruction (SVCO).

Venous thrombosis blood clot, DVT, Deep Vein Thrombosis – This is a sudden onset of asymmetrical (one sided) tense edema, which may be maybe painful or tender. There may be a dusky hue.

Heart failure – May present with very soft pitting edema, episodes of breathlessness exacerbated by lying flat, and waking breathless at night.

Cellulitis – This skin infection should be considered in all patients with erythema (redness) of the skin. It is usually warmer than the surrounding area or other limb. It may be associated with pain, and the person may feel systemically unwell or have (pyrexia) fever.

Local malignancy – This may present as demarcated cancer lesions in the skin.

Lymphedema – The limb size increases gradually. In the early stages, the edema may be soft and pit easily on pressing but does not pit easily in the later stages.

Treatment/things you can do to add comfort:

1. Focus is on skin care, limb positioning and support, massage, and containment.
2. Wash, using pH-neutral soap, carefully drying the skin.
3. Moisturize where appropriate.
4. Minimize the risk of trauma to the skin.
5. Observe skin condition for potential problems.
6. Limb positioning and support – should be elevated at level of the heart.
7. Exercise to stimulate lymphatic and venous drainage.
8. Encourage normal use and limb function.
9. Avoid excessive exercise.
10. Consider physiotherapy referral.

Skin and wounds

Itching, otherwise known as pruritus, is an irritating skin sensation causing a desire to scratch. It can be unpleasant and lead to scratching and rubbing off the skin, leading to restlessness, anxiety, skin sores, and infection. For those at moderate or high risk of pressure damage, a special mattress, seat cushion, and careful handling will reduce the risk of tissue breakdown. Adequate nutrition and hydration are important, and it is possible that stress plays a part by delaying healing. Try to eat a balanced diet, drink plenty of water, and limit stress.

Pressure ulcers, also known as pressure sores, bedsores, or decubitus ulcers, are caused by localized damage to the skin and/or underlying tissue, and usually occur over bony prominences due to pressure/shearing, or friction. The best way to approach bedsores is prevention.

*Free Bonus Material at my website, www.HomeHospice Book.com, for a link to a full-page, full-colour diagram of pressure points over bony prominences, for you to print.

Tips for overall skin health

Consider the following suggestions for skin health:

- Aim for a balanced diet, including a good protein source, and a variety of fruits and vegetables.
- Drink plenty of fluids.
- Take a multivitamin, including beta carotene, vitamin C, and zinc as prescribed by your practitioner.
- Do not take vitamins, minerals, herbal supplements, or homeopathic remedies without a physician's supervision, as they may interact with your medications or ongoing cancer treatments.
- Never apply any herb, poultice, or supplement to any open wound without physician supervision.

- Stay out of direct sunlight, and/or use UVA and UVB sunscreen. Some of your medications may make you more prone to sunburn and sun damage.

Tips for repositioning

Consider the following recommendations related to repositioning in a bed or chair:

- Shift your weight frequently. If you use a wheelchair, try shifting your weight, about every 15 minutes. Ask for help with repositioning, about once an hour.
- Lift yourself, if possible. If you have enough upper body strength, do wheelchair push ups by raising your body off the seat and pushing on the arms of the chair.
- Look into a specialty wheelchair. Some wheelchairs allow you to tilt them, which can relieve pressure. Select cushions or a mattress that relieves pressure. Use cushions or a special mattress to relieve pressure and help ensure your body is well-positioned. Do not use doughnut cushions, as they can focus pressure on surrounding tissue.
- Adjust the elevation of your bed. If your bed can be elevated at the head, raise it no more than 30 degrees. This helps prevent shearing. [28]

Tips for skin care

Consider the following suggestions for skin care:

- Keep skin clean and dry. Wash the skin with a gentle cleanser and pat dry. Do this cleansing routine regularly to limit the skin's exposure to moisture, urine, and stool.
- Protect the skin. Apply lotion to dry skin. Change bedding and clothing frequently if needed. Watch for buttons on the clothing and wrinkles in the bedding that irritate the skin.
- Inspect the skin daily. Look closely at your skin daily for warning signs of a pressure sore. [28]

When to call for help:
- If changes do not disappear after 2 days.
- The skin takes on a yellowish color (jaundice).
- Scratching is making the skin raw.
- Rash is worsening despite using treatment.
- If you notice cracked, blistered, scaly, broken, and red skin.
- Sores that are getting larger and smell foul.
- Change in color of drainage from the sore.

Skin problems

- Preventing pressure damage starts with identifying people at risk.
- Healing of pressure damage is not realistic if the prognosis is short.

- Dry skin is common and can be uncomfortable. Regularly lubricate the skin with a non-allergenic moisturizing cream.

*Free Bonus Material at my website, www.Home HospiceBook.com, for a link to the Mayo Clinic self-management of bedsores.

Urinary and sexual symptoms

Urinary tract issues

Urinary symptoms are common in advanced disease. Symptoms of a urinary tract infection may be non-specific in the neurologically impaired, and cause agitation and restlessness. Urinary problems can be caused by local cancer, or by any condition that impairs mobility or pelvic neurological function. Urinary incontinence is the involuntary leakage of urine. Studies on the general population have demonstrated that urinary incontinence is known to have an impact on a person's quality of life, and to be linked with anxiety and depression. [30]

When to call for help:
- A decrease in urine output that is not associated with end of life.
- The inability to pass urine (urinary retention).
- Symptoms of pain, foul odor, increased or decreased frequency, back pain, or blood in the urine.
- New onset of confusion or disorientation may be the first symptom of urinary tract infection.

Urinary output change

Any significant change in urinary output should be investigated. However, if it is occurring naturally at the end of life, no action is needed.

Infections

The key signs and symptoms of infection are dysuria (pain on urination), malodor (bad odour), cloudy urine, frequency and urgency of urination, urinating small amounts, back or pelvic pain, and sometimes hematuria (blood in urine). There may or may not be a fever, and often times the first symptom of a urinary tract infection is confusion. Urine should be collected, tested, and cultured to see if any bacteria can be grown and identified. The bacteria should be tested for sensitivity to antibiotic treatments. Antibiotics can be ordered to clear infection and improve comfort. At the end of life, the decision to not treat with antibiotics may be reasonable, especially if you are unable to swallow or are unresponsive.

Bleeding

It is unusual for blood loss to be severe. Palliative radiotherapy can reduce hematuria arising from a bleeding cancer in the urinary tract. Bladder irrigation with a 1% alum solution can reduce severe bleeding from the bladder.

Pain

Trigone pain at the base of the bladder may be caused by urinary catheter balloon.

Bladder pain may be due to tumor or infection.

Ureteric pain, renal colic pain in the kidneys and ureters, can be caused by kidney stones or spasm. Pain is felt in the flanks.

Urinary incontinence

The involuntary leakage of urine.

*Free Bonus Material at my website, www.HomeHospice Book.com, for more detailed information on how to manage incontinence.

Urinary retention

The inability to completely empty the bladder. This can lead to agitation, restlessness, and pain, and requires a urinary catheter to be placed.

Sexuality and intimacy

In a 2004 study on sexuality in palliative care, patients' perspectives were that emotional connections took precedence over physical expressions of sexuality. Sexuality was reported to be important to people, even at end of life. Some barriers to expressing sexuality in the hospital and the hospice setting were lack of privacy, shared rooms, staff intrusion, and the physical layout of the rooms, which mostly include single beds. [57]

Sexual dysfunction (or sexual malfunction, or sexual disorder) is the difficulty experienced by an individual or a couple during any stage of normal sexual activity, including physical pleasure, desire, preference, arousal, or orgasm. This may result from impaired body function, altered body image, or from the emotional and psychological distress that often accompanies a terminal diagnosis and treatment. [29]

Illness can often lead to changing roles and responsibilities in a relationship. These changes can be challenging during the adjustment phase. A lack of discussion can lead to feelings of distance and lack of intimacy.

Despite the many ways in which advanced disease can cause sexual dysfunction, it is uncommon for sexual problems to be discussed or explored by healthcare providers. Acknowledging and addressing any issues surrounding sexuality is an important factor in quality of life for you and your partner.

Despite the many challenges, many individuals and couples continue to enjoy a healthy sexuality, contributing to improved quality of life.

Erectile dysfunction – Erectile dysfunction (ED), also known as impotence, is a type of sexual dysfunction characterized by the inability to develop or maintain an erection of the penis during sexual activity. If erectile impotence persists, a trial of sildenafil is worthwhile, as many patients with advanced disease do not have the inclination or time to wait for a full impotence assessment.

Hormonal deficiency – In women, this can cause a loss of sexual interest. Painful intercourse because of dryness and vaginitis may be helped by lubrication or estrogen creams. In men, hormone deficiency can cause erectile dysfunction, a loss of sexual interest, and depression.

Altered body image – This can impair a person's perception of their sexuality and lead to depression.

Urinary incontinence and discharge, vaginal discharge, or bleeding due to tumor will often result in a cessation of intercourse.

Sex and the catheter – Some patients with catheters, and their partners, are still able and willing to consider intercourse, but they are afraid of the catheter. Women can have intercourse with an indwelling catheter. Intermittent self-catheterization is a better alternative. Men who are able to achieve an erection can do so with a catheter present. Gentle intercourse is possible for men with a disconnected catheter (after draining the bladder), by placing a condom over the penis and catheter. If the ejaculatory mechanism is undamaged, this can still occur with a catheter but may be painful. [27]

Maintaining intimacy – In a relationship, this does not always involve sex. Holding hands, kissing, and cuddling can be both intimate and affectionate.

Tips for maintaining intimacy with your partner

Maintain open communication by talking to your partner about your feelings regarding sex and intimacy. Find a time and place where you can both feel free to talk openly and privately.

During a terminal illness, your sexual interests and desires may change: either decreased sexual interests or, possibly, increased sexual desire may occur.

You or your partner may be fearful of causing pain or receiving pain during sexual activity. Exploring different sexual positions can avoid pain and add interest to your sex life.

Share your concerns and feelings with your partner. Working together as a team can add to feelings of greater satisfaction and intimacy.

As you have physical and emotional changes during your illness, your needs may change. It is important to maintain ongoing communication.

Physical touch plays an important role in quality of life, and is an important part of intimacy. Massage can be comforting, sexual, or therapeutic, depending on the intention.

Holding hands, kissing, and cuddling can be both intimate and affectionate.

If you are not asked directly, you can feel comfortable bringing up the topic of privacy and intimacy, with your healthcare team. You have the right to private time with your partner.

Take time to reconnect as a couple: look at old pictures, reminisce about falling in love, have a quiet meal together or, if possible, a date night.

Emotional connections can also be intimate, and include listening to music together, watching a favorite movie, sharing poetry, or just simply lying close together.

Take each day as it comes, and enjoy the time you have together; enjoy being present in each other's company.

If body changes and body image is a concern, there are resources available to help with makeovers, wigs, and accessories, to help improve self-esteem.

When to call for help:
- If you have erectile dysfunction, lack of desire, or physical discomfort during sexual intercourse, your physician may be able to investigate and offer some solutions.
- If you have emotional or psychological distress, either individual or couples counseling may be helpful.

Gastrointestinal

Oral problems

- A healthy mouth has an intact mucosa, and is clean, moist, and pain-free.
- Regular mouth care will prevent many oral problems.
- **Candidiasis** (oral thrush) and dry mouth are the two most common problems.
- **Mucositis** is the painful inflammation and ulceration of the mucous membranes lining the digestive tract, usually as a side effect of chemotherapy and radiotherapy treatment for cancer.

Maintaining oral hygiene is very important to reduce infections and treatment-induced mucositis (inflammation of oral cavity). A soft toothbrush will gently clean coated tongue and teeth, but foam sticks or gauze are less effective. Irrigation with warm water or 0.9% saline will help with removal of oral debris.

Dysphagia (difficulty swallowing)

Dysphagia is defined as difficulty or discomfort in swallowing as a symptom of disease. It is often seen in cancer, especially in the head, neck, or lung, but is more common in people with neurological diseases, such as amyotrophic lateral sclerosis (ALS), motor neurone disease (MND), stroke, multiple sclerosis, dementia, Parkinson's disease, cerebral palsy, and frailty of old age. Around 60% of people with ALS have dysphagia.

Treatment

Evaluation for a swallow assessment, by a speech and language pathologist, may be necessary.

Small portions of attractively presented foods are essential.

Dexamethasone reduces edema and can improve neurological function but may increase the risk of oral candidiasis (thrush).

Radiotherapy may be given in a single intra cavity dose.

Esophageal dilation is a procedure that allows your doctor to dilate, or stretch, a narrowed area of your esophagus [swallowing tube]. This may be effective in malignant obstruction but only last a few weeks.

Laser has advantages over intubation.

Esophageal stenting – small, expandable metal stents are placed in the esophagus to help keep the swallowing tube open.

Non-oral feeding and hydration

This may be required if you are unable to manage your nutrition requirements orally, and includes a nasogastric feeding tube (a tube that goes through your nose into your stomach, which may be tolerated poorly by most people) or percutaneous gastrostomy tube (PEG). A PEG tube is a tube that goes through your abdominal wall, straight into your stomach, and is placed with a minor surgical procedure, which is usually well tolerated.

A note on feeding and hydration at end of life:

At the end of life, hunger and thirst are not usually a problem, and unwanted feeding or hydration by any route may increase distress.

Food and fluids may be aspirated (inhaled) into the lungs and cause pneumonia.

Excess fluids, either taken by mouth or by intravenous (in a vein) or subcutaneous (under the skin) injections, may not be tolerated by the kidneys, and cause fluid to accumulate in the lungs and tissues of the body.

The best way to ensure comfort at end of life is by providing good oral mouth care.

Dyspepsia (indigestion)

Dyspepsia can be defined as painful or disturbed digestion, which may be accompanied by symptoms such as nausea and vomiting, heartburn, bloating, and stomach discomfort. Three types are now recognized: structural dyspepsia, functional dyspepsia, and gastro-esophageal reflux disease (GERD).

Treatment

Lifestyle changes, to help relieve your symptoms of dyspepsia.

Change your eating and lifestyle habits
- Eat several small meals instead of two or three large meals.
- Wait 2 to 3 hours, after you eat, before you lie down. Do not have late-night snacks.
- Avoid chocolate, mint, and alcohol, as they relax the valve between the esophagus and the stomach.
- Avoid spicy foods.
- Avoid acidic foods such as tomatoes, oranges, and coffee.
- Do not smoke or chew tobacco.
- Raise the head of your bed 6 to 8 inches by putting the frame on blocks, or by placing a foam wedge under the head of your mattress.
- Avoid wearing tight clothing around your middle.
- Losing just 5 to 10 pounds can help, if you are overweight. [71]

Medications

Avoid anti-inflammatories, such as ibuprofen, naproxen, toradol, and aspirin.

Treatment depends on what is causing the problem. If no specific cause is found, treatment with medicine focuses on relieving symptoms.

When to call for help:

Alarming symptoms would normally require prompt investigation and treatment.

- Prompts for urgent investigation: chronic gastrointestinal bleeding; unintentional weight loss; difficulty swallowing; persistent vomiting; iron deficiency anemia.
- Prompts for immediate investigation and management: Rapid clinical deterioration; persistent vomiting, causing dehydration; electrolyte disturbance; hematemesis (from bleeding ulcer or severe gastritis); melena dark stools (upper gastrointestinal hemorrhage); persistent and worsening pain (perforation or other intra-abdominal crisis); severe difficulty swallowing (esophageal obstruction).

Nausea and vomiting

Nausea and vomiting occurs in up to 50% of patients with cancer, and both are common in AIDS, end-stage heart failure, and in children at the end of life.

Choosing an antiemetic (anti-nausea)

These are dimenhydrinate, haloperidol, metoclopramide, domperidone, and methotrimrprazine.

Associated management

Bucket, tissues, and water: A decent sized bowl is essential to avoid the distress to patients of soiling their clothes and bedsheets. Also available should be tissues to wipe the mouth, and water or juice to rinse the mouth.

Parenteral (non-oral) hydration, either intravenous or subcutaneous, and nasogastric tube and suction, has no role to play in most causes of nausea and vomiting.

Acupuncture has good evidence for efficacy with nausea and vomiting.

Acupressure at the P6 acupuncture point on the wrist may have a role in some patients.

Chemotherapy is only helpful in treating nausea and vomiting if there is likely to be a good tumor response.

Hypnosis and behavioral therapy can be helpful.

Disorders of the bowels

Common names
Bowel movements, BM, diarrhea, faeces, feces, poop, poo, shit, stool.

Incontinence

Incontinence of the bowel or bladder can be an embarrassing and overwhelming problem to deal with, for everyone involved.

*Free Bonus Material at my website, www.HomeHospice Book.com, for more detailed information on how to manage incontinence.

Diarrhea

- Oral rehydration is an essential part of management.
- Infection should be excluded, with a stool sample being sent to the lab for culture.
- Constipation with overflow can be a cause.

Diarrhea is a condition in which feces are discharged from the bowels frequently, and in a liquid form, and is also classified into acute, which lasts one or two weeks, and chronic, which continues for longer than 2 or 3 weeks. Viral and bacterial infections are the most common causes of acute diarrhea. It occurs in up to 10% of cancer patients, and up to 38% of people with AIDS. It is exhausting and distressing. Fecal incontinence can create a loss of dignity for you, and high stress for your loved ones. Risk factors for fecal incontinence include advancing age, immobility, neurological disease, spinal injury, previous obstetric trauma, pelvic prolapse, previous colonic or rectal surgery, hospitalized patients, diabetes, fecal impaction, stroke, and severe cognitive impairment.

*Free Bonus Material at my website, www.HomeHospice Book.com

When to call for help:
Mild dehydration
Thirst, reduced urine output, reduced skin elasticity.
Severe dehydration (clinical shock)
Decreased or altered level of consciousness, delirium, pale or mottled skin, cold limbs, weak pulse, fast heart rate, and fast breathing.

Treatment

Rehydration: For adults, rehydration powders offered no advantages for those able to maintain oral intake.

Medication: Your physician may prescribe loperamide, an antidiarrheal medication.

Constipation

Constipation is a condition in which there is difficulty in emptying the bowels. It is usually associated with hardened feces, and is a common and distressing problem in cancer, AIDS, cardiac disease, respiratory disease, and adrenal disease. It is often due to pain medications, but it can be caused by many other drugs, as well as biochemical abnormalities, such as hypercalcemia (high calcium), and metabolic problems, such as diabetes.

Definition

Constipation is the passage of small, hard feces, infrequently and with difficulty, usually accompanied by additional symptoms. Constipation is a common cause of distress and may increase agitation and confusion, or precipitate seizures in children.

Symptoms:

Reduced frequency of stool is common in advanced disease. Abdominal pain, flatulence, abdominal distention, nausea, vomiting, halitosis (bad breath), overflow diarrhea, malaise, fecal incontinence, anorexia (decreased appetite).

It is important to monitor the bowels daily. You may likely need to take a stool softener and a stimulant laxative on a routine basis, if you are taking opioid narcotic medications.

It is important understand that you need both a soft stool and a contracting bowel in order to have regular bowel movements.

You may need a rectal stimulant, such as a suppository or enema, especially if there are some neurological issues.

Let your health care provider know if you have not had a bowel movement in two days.

For more detailed information on managing the bowels, and to access a stool chart, you can access my website at www.HomeHospiceBook.com.

All laxatives and rectal measures have a delay before they act, and their effect can be assessed. [27]

Rectal measures:	Time to Effect
docusate enema	5–20 min
bisacodyl suppository	15–60 min
glycerine suppository	15–60 min
arachis oil enema	1 hour
Injectable opioid reversal agent:	
methylnaltrexone SC	20 min–4 hours
Contact stimulants (oral)	
sennosides	8–12 hours
bisacodyl	6–12 hours
Softening laxatives (oral)	
lactulose	1–2 days
docusate	1–3 days
macrogols	1–3 days

Diet and exercise

One study showed, to achieve a 50% increase in bowel frequency, a person would have to take over four times as much fiber. The correlation between activity and exercise is weak. [27]

Ascites

Ascites is the accumulation of fluid in the peritoneal cavity, causing abdominal swelling, nausea, vomiting, abdominal distention or pain, edema (legs, perineum for lower trunk), and breathlessness due to diaphragmatic splinting.

Treatment

Diuretics (water pills), paracentesis (drainage of the fluid by a procedure), and peritoneal-venous shunting are still the mainstay of treatment, although the evidence for all three is weak.

Bowel obstruction

Intestinal obstruction is a blockage that keeps food or liquid from passing through your small intestine or large intestine (colon). It can be a dramatic and frightening development but is not always terminal. Medical management will keep the majority of people comfortable and free of nausea and pain, allowing them to remain at home.

Causes of bowel obstruction
- Gastrointestinal cancers
- Obstruction from tumors
- Constipation
- Benign adhesions may occur in up to 20% of people with abdominal cancer, previous surgery, or radiotherapy.
- Motility disorders, causing a physical blockage

Treatment options
- Surgery should always be considered.
- Stents can be an option in patients unable to have surgery.
- Nasogastric tube is generally ineffective.
- Gastrostomy or jejunostomy tubes may be appropriate for persistent vomiting.

Medical management
- Medications
- Bowel rest
- Hydration (intravenous or subcutaneous hypodermaclysis)

Suggestions for things you can do to bring comfort and dignity
- Create a safe place to express suffering: one that enables you and family to feel safe to express your distress.
- Ensure you are at the center of treatment decisions.
- Do not wait for your loved one to complain about symptoms; you can ask and observe.
- Do not delay starting treatment. Symptoms should be treated promptly, since they become more difficult to treat, the longer they are left.

- Administer drugs regularly, in doses titrated to each individual, to ensure the symptom does not return.
- Set realistic goals. Negotiate some additional shorter-term goals.
- Reassess repeatedly and regularly. Treat concurrent symptoms. People with other symptoms, such as nausea and breathlessness, experience more pain than those without these symptoms.
- Sympathy, understanding, diversion, and elevation of mood are essential adjuncts.
- Encourage bed rest, with feet up on two pillows if there is swelling.
- Remove rings and jewelry before they become too tight.
- A soft toothbrush will gently clean coated tongue and teeth, but foam sticks or gauze are less effective.
- Irrigation with warm water or 0.9% saline will help removal of oral debris.
- For vomiting, have a bucket, tissues, and water: A decent sized bowl is essential to avoid the distress to patients of soiling their clothes and bedsheets. Also available should be tissues to wipe the mouth, and water or juice to rinse the mouth.
- To avoid constipation, get appropriate laxatives regularly, and titrate to maintain a comfortable stool.
- Increase fiber and fluid to help with constipation.
- Patients with colostomies: inserting a gloved finger will show if feces are present.

My notes, thoughts, questions, and next chapter

I highly recommend that you write down any ideas, questions, thoughts, and reflections that may be important to you. Please feel free to use your book as a companion on this, your journey, and take your book with questions to your care providers to help start those difficult conversations.

In this chapter of *The Book on Home Hospice,* you have gained some knowledge about the many physical symptoms that can be common, and cause you distress. This chapter has given you some ideas and tips for alleviating symptoms of suffering for yourself or your loved one, and to help you to be comfortable while you are at home. Read the next chapter on medical emergencies for some very important information to help you recognize and report symptoms of opioid toxicity, opioid overdose, bleeding, convulsions, superior vena cava syndrome, and spinal cord compression.

For more detailed information, you can access my website at www.HomeHospiceBook.com.

Notes

Chapter 5
Medical Emergencies

Keep Calm and Carry On

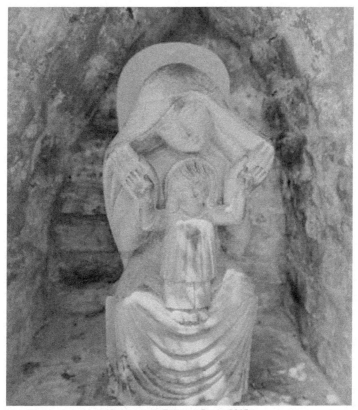

Photo.credit:Deborah.Dooler2017

In this very important chapter of *The Book on Home Hospice,* it will be essential for you to know how to recognize and respond to rare but important medical emergencies in the home. The topics covered will be opioid toxicity, opioid overdose, bleeding, convulsions, superior vena cava syndrome, and spinal cord compression. During the transition towards the end of life, your body may change suddenly due to some rare but serious complications. These sudden changes can be frightening for you and your family, but recognizing what signs and symptoms to look for, and what you can do to help, can be reassuring.

Important
Call your home care nurse or physician, or call 911 emergency services immediately, if you are concerned.

Opioid toxicity

Opioid toxicity occurs when taking narcotic medications such as morphine, hydromorphone, hydrocodone, oxycodone, fentanyl, tramadol, and methadone. Over time, the body may have an accumulation of toxins that the liver and kidneys are not able to release. This may lead to physical and behavioral changes.

Report any concerns or changes to your
home care nurse or physician. Or call 911.

Changes to watch for and report:
Delirium, confusion, agitation, bad dreams, decreased level of consciousness, restlessness, short-term jerking or seizure-like movements, seizures, or pain when touched, even gently.

Opioid overdose

Opioid narcotic overdose can cause death, and can be intentional or unintentional. The amount of opioid a person needs is dependent upon their body size and tolerance, which is how much their body is used to taking. Effects of an overdose can appear if the medication is given too quickly or in too large of a dose, or the body is unable to process the medication due to liver or kidney failure.

Opioid overdose can be treated with a medication called naloxone (Narcan). [36]

Report any concerns, or changes, to your
home care nurse or physician. Or call 911.

Changes to watch for and report:
- The person can become tired, stop talking, or become unresponsive.
- Breathing remains regular but becomes very slow; it may drop to less than six breaths per minute and may even stop. This is a medical emergency.

Bleeding

Severe hemorrhage

Hemorrhage, also known as exsanguination, is defined as an escape of blood from a ruptured blood vessel. Since small, repeated bleeds can herald a major bleed, hemorrhage is a common fear. In reality, death from hemorrhage is rare. It can be more common with stomach and bowel tumors, or tumors that are close to major arteries.

In any setting, use dark green, blue, or black towels to soak up the blood loss, as the absorbed blood will appear a less frightening black, and not red. Perineal pads will help with the management of vaginal and low gastrointestinal bleeding. You will feel cold because of the hypotension (low blood pressure), and will need warm blankets. Such an event is frightening for all involved, and your palliative care team, or a family physician, should have a plan in place in the unlikely event of a catastrophic bleed, if you have a high-risk condition. [27] It is important to recognize that bleeding may be external or internal.

Sedative medications, such as midazolam, may be used for comfort.

Report any concerns about bleeding to your home care nurse or physician immediately. Or call 911.

Changes to watch for and report:
- Bleeding from a tumor, the mouth, ears, nose, bowels, urinary tract, or vagina.
- Internal bleeding will cause symptoms of shock, pale clammy skin, decreased levels of consciousness, rapid heart rate, and low blood pressure.
- Internal bleeding can also occur around and in the brain. This may start as a headache, described as the worst headache of your life. It can lead to a decreased level of consciousness and death.
- There may or may not be bruising.

Convulsions

A convulsion or seizure is defined as a sudden, violent, irregular movement of a limb or of the body, caused by involuntary contraction of muscles, and is especially associated with brain disorders, such as epilepsy and brain tumors, or the presence of certain toxins or other agents in the blood, or fever in children. Although convulsions can be frightening, they generally will stop on their own after a few seconds or minutes.

Report any concerns to your home care nurse
or physician immediately. Or call 911.

Changes to watch for and report:
- A seizure lasting more than 5 minutes.
- The person does not regain consciousness.
- First seizure.

Superior vena cava syndrome

Superior vena cava syndrome (SVCS) is a group of symptoms caused by obstruction of the superior vena cava (a short, wide vessel carrying circulating blood into the heart from the body). More than 90% of cases of superior vena cava obstruction (SVCO) are caused by cancer.

Call your physician or home care nurse
immediately so they may assess. Or call 911.

Changes to watch for and report:
Early signs:
Shortness of breath, rapid breathing, rapid heart rate, headache, standing out of neck and chest veins, and redness of face, neck, or upper trunk.
Later signs:
Swelling of the face and around the eyes, chest pain, tightness in throat, cough, difficulty with vision, and arm swelling.

Spinal cord compression

Spinal cord compression develops when the spinal cord is compressed by bone fragments from a vertebral fracture, a tumor, abscess, ruptured intervertebral disc, or another lesion. It is a medical emergency and, if left untreated, it can lead to paralysis. Approximately 5% of people with cancer will develop a cord compression.

***Report any symptoms to your home care nurse
or physician immediately. Or call 911.***

Changes to watch for and report:
Early signs:
Back pain.
Later signs:
Numbness, tingling, pins and needles, hot and cold in the limbs.
Bowel and bladder changes, incontinence, or problems passing urine and stool.
Motor changes, weakness, loss of strength.
Frequent falls.

****Free Bonus Material at my website, www.HomeHospice
Book.com***

My notes, thoughts, questions, and next chapter

I highly recommend that you write down any ideas, questions, thoughts, and reflections that may be important to you. Please feel free to use your book as a companion on this, your journey, and take your book with questions to your care providers to help start those difficult conversations.

Now that you know about some of the rare but serious medical emergencies that may occur, you will be able to recognize the signs and symptoms, and report them.

Call your home care nurse or physician, or call 911 emergency services immediately, if you are concerned.

In the chapter that follows, you will look at some of the emotional factors involved in suffering, including depression, anxiety, agitation, and insomnia, and you will learn some coping strategies to help you maintain comfort and dignity at home.

Notes

_____

_____

_____

_____

_____

_____

_____

_____

_____

_____

_____

_____

_____

_____

_____

_____

_____

_____

_____

_____

_____

_____

_____

_____

_____

Notes

Chapter 6
Relief of Common Symptoms of the Mind

The most luxurious possession, the richest treasure
anybody has, is his personal dignity.
Jackie Robinson

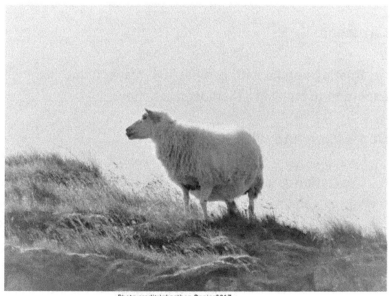

Photo.credit:Johnathon.Dooler2017

How to recognize and relieve emotional suffering

Psychological distress is a major cause of suffering in people with an advanced, life-threatening illness, and is associated with decreased quality of life and loss of dignity. More than 60% of people with cancer report experiencing distress, which can erode physical, psychological, social, and spiritual well-being. [34] This chapter in *The Book on Home Hospice* will address some of the emotional factors you may experience, including depression, anxiety, agitation, and insomnia. You will learn how to recognize the signs and symptoms, and when to report these to your palliative nurse or physician. You will acquire some strategies to help with coping with stress and maintaining dignity.

Care tenor

Treating people with compassion, respect, and dignity, is important to building a therapeutic relationship.

Depression and withdrawal

Depression is a mood disorder that causes a persistent feeling of sadness and loss of interest (also called major depressive disorder or clinical depression). You may have feelings of severe despondency and dejection. At the end of life, depression can be easily misinterpreted as sadness, or can be masked by anxiety. The usual screening tools for depression are not ideal in the setting of terminal illness.

The diagnosis of depression is made on the following characteristics:
- A persistent feeling of depressed mood, longer than 2 weeks and greater than 50% of the time.
- Change in the usual mood.
- Loss of interest and enjoyment in activities (anhedonia).
- Three or more of the following depressive related symptoms:
- Varying mood, early morning wakening, impaired concentration, feelings of hopelessness, guilt, shame, feeling a burden to others, thoughts of self-harm, desire to hasten death, loss of energy, change in appetite, and change in sex drive. [27]

Treatment options

There is little research on treating depression in advanced disease; however, depression should be treated, if present. [27] Depression is a treatable illness, even in the seriously ill person. Treating depression may alleviate both physical and psychological suffering of both the person and caregivers. [34]

- Antidepressant medications should be considered, even at end of life, depending on prognosis.
- Cognitive behavioral therapy (CBT) may be helpful.
- Patient and family supportive psychotherapy may be helpful.
- Psychiatric referral may be appropriate in some cases. [34]

Depression and caregivers

Several studies have examined the relationship between patient and caregivers' depressive symptoms. Depressive symptoms in caregivers are common, and correlate with the lack of responsiveness of their loved ones to depression treatment. A family-oriented response to depression may be helpful. [34]

Withdrawal from the external world

As the end of life approaches, there is a feeling of detachment from the physical world, and a loss of interest in things you formerly found pleasurable. There is a tendency to sleep more. There is less desire to talk. This is the beginning of letting go of life, and preparing for death. [35]

Dignity therapy

A therapeutic intervention targets depression and suffering, and enhances a sense of meaning and purpose at the end of life. It allows people to address grief-related issues, offers comfort to loved ones, and provides instructions to friends and families on how to recall meaningful, personal history.

Anxiety

Anxiety disorders are the most common psychiatric disorder in the general population, with up to 29% prevalence [34]; and symptoms of anxiety can occur in greater than 70% of medically ill people, especially those with cancer, approaching end of life. [34]

Anxiety is defined as an expected, transient response to stress, and can result in a feeling of worry, nervousness, or unease, typically about an imminent event, or something with an uncertain outcome. Normal anxiety is a protective mechanism for times of danger and stress. Pathological, or abnormal anxiety, is an excessive response to external or internal stress. [34]

Anxiety is an emotion characterized by an unpleasant state of inner turmoil, often accompanied by nervous behavior, such as pacing back and forth, or having somatic complaints, such as physical sensations. Some examples include pain, nausea, dizziness, fainting, and rumination (thinking about the same thing over and over again). You can have unpleasant feelings of dread over anticipated events, such as the feeling of imminent death. [27] Life-threatening illness creates an uncertain future that causes anxiety, which may increase as the illness progresses. Anxiety, in turn, makes it more difficult for you to cope with suffering.

Identifying anxiety

Features of anxiety are:

Apprehensive expectation – Fear, and tendency to perceive situations in a threatening way.

Rumination – To go over a thought in the mind, repeatedly and often.

Vigilance – The action or state of keeping careful watch for possible danger or difficulties.

Scanning – Irritability, poor concentration, difficulty getting to sleep, tendency to perceive bodily sensations in a threatening way.

Motor tension – Trembling, tension, restlessness.

Autonomic hyperactivity – Sweating, dry mouth, cold hands, tachycardia (fast heart beat), diarrhea.

Depression – In advanced disease, anxiety is often associated with depressed mood. [27]

Treatment options
- Anxiety is common in advanced disease, and symptoms should be treated with medication.
- Anxiety can be eased with clear communication and simple measures.
- Anxiety and depression often coexist and should be treated concurrently.
- Cognitive behavioral therapy (CBT) may be helpful.
- Patient and family supportive psychotherapy may be helpful.
- Psychiatric referral may be appropriate in some cases of severe anxiety.

Helping the anxious person

Supportive measures:
- Enabling a person to express their feelings, to discuss their needs and fears about the end of life, to give the information they need, can do much to ease anxiety and maintain dignity.
- Identify the triggers for anxiety.
- Evidence for reflexology in treating anxiety is conflicting.
- Complementary approaches include hypnosis, music therapy, and aromatherapy.
- Moderate anxiety will ease with anxiety suppressants, such as Lorazepam, which is effective in low doses, with little sedation.
- Severe anxiety will require antipsychotics.

Panic: This occurs suddenly, without an obvious cause, is intense, and can last 5 to 20 minutes. A fear of dying and loss of control is felt with panic attacks.

Phobias: An irrational fear of an object or situation, and may respond to cognitive behavioral therapy (CBT) or medications.

Agitation, delirium, confusion

Delirium is defined as an acutely disturbed state of mind that occurs in fever, intoxication, and other disorders, and is characterized by restlessness, illusions, and incoherence of thought and speech. It is extremely common among people who are hospitalized or are in a nursing home, with studies to suggest anywhere from 30 to 50%, and has been reported up to as much as 88%, of people near the end of life. [34] At the end of life, acute confusion can go hand-in-hand with physical illnesses, and can lead to suffering and loss of dignity. Delirium significantly contributes to caregiver burden and the inability to cope at home.

Diagnosing confusional states

Acute confusional state (delirium)
Four features are typical of delirium:
- Acute onset, and fluctuating (changing) course.
- Inattention.
- Disorganized thinking.
- Altered level of alertness.

Chronic confusional state (dementia)
Can appear similar to delirium, but with the history of years:
- Symptoms that fluctuate less.
- Alertness is unlikely to have changed.

Identifying delirium

The most common causes of delirium:
Drugs, kidney and/or liver failure, low oxygen, infection, high calcium level, dehydration, low glucose, urinary retention, and constipation.

Treatment options
- Identify and treat the underlying cause.
- Treatment should be taken with the care goals clearly defined.
- Distressing symptoms should be managed with appropriate antipsychotic or sedative medications.
- Family supportive therapy.

Non-medical interventions for delirium treatment:
- Frequent orientation (familiar objects, pictures, introductions, orientation board).
- Cognitive brain exercises.
- Oral rehydration can be achieved by having a drink available within reach, with frequent prompting to drink.
- Attention to your lighting – use natural lighting during the day and dim lighting at night.
- Sensory aides, such as glasses and hearing aids.
- Consistent caregivers.
- To help with sleep, use warm milk or herbal tea, relaxation tapes or music, and massage.
- Keep to a daily routine.
- Range of motion or physical activity.
- Limit the use of immobilization by limiting the use of Foley catheter, intravenous line, and restraints. [34]

Free Bonus Material at my website, www.HomeHospice Book.com

Insomnia

Studies conclude that insomnia is a common symptom in terminally ill people, with up to as many as 70% of people reporting insomnia at end of life [33]. Insomnia, also known as sleeplessness, is a sleep disorder where people have trouble sleeping. You may have difficulty falling asleep, or staying asleep as long as desired. Insomnia is typically followed by daytime sleepiness, low energy, irritability, and a depressed mood.

Insomnia can be caused by anxiety, fear, sadness, or other psychological or spiritual concerns. It can also be aggravated by physical symptoms such as pain, nausea, vomiting, or coughing.

Sleep at night can be disrupted by daytime naps and drowsiness.

Speak to your palliative care nurse or physician to assess for the need of medications that can help you sleep.

Some suggestions to help with sleep:
- Sleep at any time you are tired; do not follow a schedule.
- Drink warm, non-caffeinated drinks before bed.
- Spend quiet time before bedtime by reading or listening to music.
- Back massages or foot rubs can be helpful for relaxation.
- Keep the area quiet for sleeping.

When to call for help:
- If there are concerns that the person is a danger to himself or others (suicide or homicide).
- Worsening of agitation or confusion occurs suddenly.
- Violence or aggression.
- Someone is injured.
- You need relief due to exhaustion.

My notes, thoughts, questions, and next chapter

I highly recommend that you write down any ideas, questions, thoughts, and reflections that may be important to you. Please feel free to use your book as a companion on this, your journey, and take your book with questions to your care providers to help start those difficult conversations.

This chapter has taught you how to recognize and manage some of the common emotional and psychological issues that you may face. The next chapter in *The Book of Home Hospice* will continue to expand on the emotional and spiritual connection, while focusing on quality of life and living life to the fullest. It will discuss complementary and alternative therapies, spirituality, religion, community support services, legacy work, and mindfulness.

Notes

Chapter 7
Quality of Life – Living Life to the Fullest

The meaning of life is to find **Bliss.**

My mission in this lifetime is to:

B- Be happy

L- Love and be loved

I- Inspire and be inspired

S- Share joy

S- Soar higher than I thought I ever could

To live my life until I have no more life to live.

Dr. Deborah Dooler

Founder and CEO of the Dooler Institute

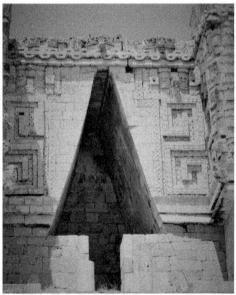

Photo.credit:Deborah.Dooler2017

In this chapter in *The Book of Home Hospice,* I will be exploring more in depth the idea of improving quality of life. There has been research looking at quality of life indicators (QOL) at the end of life (EOL). Studies have shown that people who died at home had significantly better QOL than those who died in intensive care units and hospital wards. [65] In this chapter, you will learn how alternative therapies, spirituality, religion, community support services, and mindfulness practices can be beneficial in improving how you feel physically, emotionally, and spiritually.

One study of advanced cancer patients who were dying, looked at quality of life indicators, and found that those people who avoided hospitalization and intensive care, who were not worried, who pray or meditate, who are visited by a pastor, and feel a therapeutic alliance with their physician, had the highest quality of life scores at end of life. [65] Another large study looked at complementary and alternative medicine in cancer pain management, and its impact on improving quality of life. [64] It is important to choose reputable and accredited sources for any complementary, alternative, or mindfulness therapies. A good starting place for resources include local hospices and local Wellspring organizations.

Complementary and alternative therapies

Aboriginal traditional healing – This is used to describe a broad array of traditional healing methods used by aboriginal peoples for thousands of years. There is a focus on spiritual, mental, emotional, and physical healing. It may include the medicine wheel, and sacred herbs such as tobacco, sweet grass, cedar, and sage. Traditional aboriginal healers may use methods such as sweats, smudging, healing circles, ceremonies, traditional diets, and herbal medicines.

Some research evidence suggests aboriginal traditional healings offer psychosocial, emotional, and spiritual support, and offer a feeling of powerful connection to community and the Earth, thereby decreasing stress, anxiety, and depression. [70]

Chiropractic therapy – Chiropractic therapy is most commonly used to treat back and neck pain, headache, muscle, and joint problems. A hands-on manipulation may be used, and may include heat and cold, ultrasound, electrical stimulation, massage, and traction. According to the Canadian Cancer Society, there are no available research studies verifying the benefits of chiropractic therapy in the cancer population. If working with a chiropractor, it is important to let him or her know that you have cancer. [70]

Chiropractic Doctors (CD) are regulated by the Canadian Federation of Chiropractic Regulatory and Educational Accrediting Board. It is important to only be treated by regulated professionals.

Important notice
Chiropractic therapies may not be recommended due to the risks associated with it if you have bone cancer, leukemia, multiple myeloma, certain breast or prostate cancers, osteoporosis, problems with bleeding, or stroke. Always check with your healthcare team prior to any chiropractic treatments.
Chiropractic manipulation is thought to be safe; however, there have been rare examples of stroke caused by neck manipulation. [70]

Herbal remedies include the use of special diets and enemas, and herbal, vitamin, and mineral remedies. Naturopathic medicine, homeopathic medicine, and traditional Chinese herbal medicine are commonly used herbal remedies. [70]

Naturopathic doctors (ND) are regulated in Canada, and require a full-time, three-year training program. It is important to be aware that some people call themselves a naturopath but have not been trained as a naturopathic doctor. Naturopathic medicine uses a holistic approach to support the body's own ability to heal itself, including lifestyle and diet modification. [70] This may include homeopathy, acupuncture, massage therapy, and other remedies.

Homeopathic medicine – Practitioners may have many different levels of education and training. In Canada, homeopaths are regulated in Ontario only, by the College of Homeopaths. Homeopathy is a healing system that uses remedies that are highly diluted and usually given in pill form. Remedies are chosen to reverse disharmony in the body.

Traditional Chinese herbal medicine has been used in China for thousands of years, and is often used in conjunction with acupuncture, massage, and Tai Chi. Many research studies have been reported in Chinese language journals, and it's difficult to endorse the safety of the remedies, especially alongside traditional chemotherapy medications and radiation therapy.

Some traditional Chinese herbal remedies may interact with other medications, over-the-counter and herbs, and may be dangerous to your health. [70]

Caution
Any herbal remedy should be taken with caution, and the healthcare team, family physician, palliative physician, oncology, and specialty physicians should be aware of what you are taking, as there is a risk of interaction with conventional medications and treatments, such as chemotherapy and radiation therapy.

Energy therapies are used to manipulate the flow of energy through the body, and include Reiki, therapeutic touch, healing touch, and magnetic healing therapy. Some studies have shown reports of improvement in quality of life; there is little evidence to show a change in energy flow. Energy therapies are thought to be safe, with few side effects. [70]

Reiki – Practitioners believe channeling spiritual energy through their hands can help healing.

Therapeutic touch – Practitioners move their hands just above the body to remove harmful energy, replacing it with healthy energy.

Healing touch – Gentle touch is used to heal energy fields.

Magnetic healing therapy – Magnets are used on the body to unblock energy flow.

The Emotional Freedom Technique (EFT) – Also known as *Tapping Therapy* or *Meridian Tapping Techniques* (MTT), it was created by Gary Craig, and works like emotional acupressure to quickly, gently, and easily release the negative emotions and beliefs that are at the root of all our problems and pain.

Peripheral therapy involves stimulating the skin, and includes hot and cold treatments, exercise such as yoga and Tai Chi, acupuncture, hydrotherapy (water therapy), transcutaneous electrical nerve stimulation (TENS), massage therapy, and therapeutic touch, including Reiki and reflexology. These are believed to be helpful with inflammation swelling and muscle spasm. [64]

Yoga is an ancient healing system using exercise, breathing, and meditation to align your energy. Yoga has been found in some studies to improve quality of life, and to be beneficial in managing symptoms such as fatigue, anxiety, and mood, although there is little evidence to support a great improvement in pain. [64]

Tai Chi is an ancient, Chinese, healing martial art, which includes slow exercises to support the life force energy. Studies have shown that Tai Chi can significantly improve exercise capacity, muscle strength, and flexibility, as well as improved quality of life indicators. [64]

Acupuncture is a traditional Chinese medicine technique that uses needles applied by a specially trained professional to specific points on the body, and has shown evidence in relieving nausea and vomiting, pain and stiffness, hot flashes, and fatigue. There is evidence showing effective pain control, although more research is needed into the ability of applying acupuncture in the home setting. [64]

Transcutaneous electrical nerve stimulation (TENS) is a unit that delivers low voltage electricity to leads placed over the skin near the painful site. Mixed results have been found for chronic cancer pain; however, for mild pain, there may be a benefit from TENS. It should be only initiated by a professional, as electrodes can be dangerous if placed in the wrong areas, such as near the eyes, the neck, open wounds, infections, and tumors, or in pregnant women, and on the genitals. It is dangerous to use on people with a pacemaker or cardiac defibrillator, or on those with epilepsy or undiagnosed pain. [64]

Massage therapy involves hands-on manual techniques that are applied to the muscles and soft tissues of the body. Studies have shown massage therapy improved quality of life by increasing well-being, reducing stress and anxiety, and improving pain control. There is no evidence that massage therapy can cure cancer. [64]

Manual lymph drainage is a specialized massage therapy used to treat lymphedema, along with complex decongestive therapy, which includes compression garments; exercises and skincare can relieve symptoms. [64]

Reflexology is the use of manual pressure applied to specific areas of the body—for example, feet, hands, or ears—that are believed to correspond with other areas of the body or organs. There's a lack of medical data; however, patients have reported an improvement of their symptoms. Reflexology does not appear to be dangerous. [64]

Cognitive therapies use the mind and brain, and include hypnotherapy, cognitive behavioral therapies, and guided imagery.

Hypnotherapy, also known as hypnosis, is the induction of a trance-like state and suggestion to the subconscious mind that introduces behavioral changes. Hypnosis studies have shown to have a significant impact on pain, nausea, and vomiting. There is good evidence to support hypnotherapy for various procedures to decrease pain and anxiety, but inconclusive evidence for chronic pain. [64]

Cognitive behavioral therapy is a commonly used psychological treatment, and is a short-term therapy that teaches a practical approach to behavior change and problem solving.

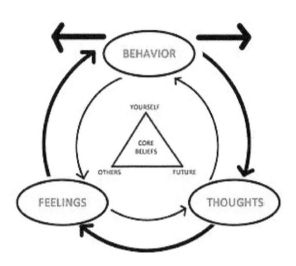

It often involves three steps:

1. Education on your thoughts, feelings, and behaviors and coping mechanisms, and how they relate to your core beliefs.

2. Training in coping management skills (e.g., relaxation, attention diversion, active coping, passive coping, imagery, and self-calming techniques).

3. Training in home practice application of the skills.

Studies have shown that CBT is effective for short-term and medium-term management of depression and anxiety, and can improve quality of life. More research is needed in the long-term effects of CBT. [64]

Brief cognitive behavioral therapy is usually 6 to 8 sessions that include education and coping mechanisms, such as symptom diaries. Review of studies shows that 50% had positive results, suggesting that more ongoing support and therapies are more successful. [64]

Imagery and self-hypnosis based cognitive behavioral therapy involves the teaching of self-guided images, a pleasant scene allowing for diversion away from symptoms. There are some studies that show promising results. [64]

Sensory Therapies – Stimulating the senses can be helpful in causing a distraction from symptoms, thereby improving mood and relaxation. Some common therapies are Snoezelen®, a multi-sensory therapy, aromatherapy, and music therapy.

Multi-sensory stimulation therapy – Snoezelen® is a combination of two Dutch verbs: snuffelen, meaning to explore, and doezelen, meaning to relax. Snoezelen® is a registered trademark of Rompa, Chesterfield, England. It involves stimulating the senses to help interact with long-term care, with dementia or verbal communication skills at end of life. Research shows both patients and families benefiting from utilizing this experience. [66] [67]

Aromatherapy is the use of plant essences (essential oils) applied to the skin, added to the bath, or inhaled with a steamer. It is thought that aromatic oils reach the lymph system and have an effect on intercellular fluids. Studies have shown that aromatherapy essential oils are beneficial in the short term to reduce anxiety, pain, and depression, and improve sleep and wellbeing. Essential oils should be used in low dosage, and should be adopted by an aroma therapist specialist, trained in researched, evidence-based treatments. It is advised to use researched oils and not to use unfamiliar oils.

Various oils that have been found useful are syzigium aromaticum (clove), cupressus sempervirens (cypress), and pelargonium graveolens (geranium). Lavender and citrus oils of a good quality are also useful for relieving stress. [64]

Music therapy – Research has shown that music therapy was successful in decreasing symptoms, such as nausea and vomiting, in the short term. Music-based interventions have evidence to support a positive impact on pain, anxiety, mood, and quality of life.

A new area of research, called music thanatology, is being implemented as an end-of-life measure; however, there remains a limited number of studies in this area. [64]

"Music touches every part of us—our bodies, minds, relationships, and souls—and makes a difference in our quality of life, quality of care, and well-being." – Music Care, training caregivers in the therapeutic use of music.

*Free Bonus Material at my website, www.HomeHospice Book.com

Use caution with complementary and alternative therapies:

Complementary and alternative therapies that make claims promising cures for cancer, have personal stories of miracles but no scientific evidence, and are offered only at one clinic or by one person, should be avoided, as they may be dangerous or unethical.

If it seems too good to be true, it usually is.

The Canadian Cancer Society is a good resource for information regarding complementary and alternative therapies.

The American Cancer Society have a good link to information regarding complementary and alternative therapies.

Mindfulness practice

Sages, Yogis, and Zen Masters from around the world have been exploring mindfulness for thousands of years. The practice of mindfulness and meditation allows you to make time in your life for stillness, and gives you an opportunity for letting go of anything that may be holding you back from obtaining peace. The practice of yoga and Tai Chi are another way of bringing awareness by moving your body. [59] There is scientific evidence of the benefits of living in the present. Being present makes you more productive and happier. Expressions such as "live in the moment," and "carpe diem (seize the day)," are backed up with research. [63]

Mindfulness is the psychological process of bringing one's attention to experiences occurring in the present moment, which can be developed through the practice of meditation. The term *mindfulness* is a translation of the Pali term, sati, and is a significant element of Buddhist traditions. Mindfulness is an ancient Buddhist practice that aims to pay attention to the present moment. It is a spiritual framework and not associated with religion. [59] Mindfulness requires effort and discipline.

Meditation is a practice that helps to quiet the mind, and helps you become aware of yourself by stopping and being present in the moment. [59] It serves as a focus for your attention; if your mind wanders, you can bring your focus back to your breath. There are many different forms and types of meditation practices.

Meditation can be performed in many positions.

Sitting meditation – Take your seat to meditate on a cushion or chair. The sitting posture represents dignity; sit up straight with strong posture.

Walking meditation – Focus on the walking and the breathing.

Standing meditation – Learn your posture from the trees. Stand close to a tree.

Lying meditation – It is very relaxing if you can keep from falling asleep.

5 reasons to practice mindfulness
1. **Understand your pain** – Mindfulness and meditation can help you re-frame your experience of pain.
2. **Connect better** – Mindfulness helps you to give your full attention to the important people in your life.
3. **Lower stress** – Mindfulness decreases stress.
4. **Focus your mind** – Mindfulness increases your ability to focus and concentrate.
5. **Reduce brain chatter** – Mindfulness gives you a chance to clear your thoughts. [73]

My religion is kindness.
The Dalai Lama

Be kind to yourself

Loving kindness meditation – Begin with yourself; bring your attention to being kind and loving to yourself. Find a feeling of peacefulness and acceptance of yourself. Offer yourself forgiveness and love.

First, love yourself. Then, extend the love and kindness to others. Begin with your close family; extend your kindness and love to them.

Next, direct your love and kindness to anyone, or the whole world and planet.

Don't underestimate the power of doing nothing.
Winnie the Pooh

The benefits of calm

Managing your energy has the benefits of calming your brain and body. Worry and catastrophizing is exhausting, and can cause fatigue and increased stress levels. It can trick your body to go into a fight or flight mode, and it expends a lot of energy. Calm is the key to energy conservation. Structured idleness means to schedule time in your day to do nothing. [63]

Ways to create calm
- Lie down and take a break
- Relaxation
- Meditation
- Massage therapy
- Talk to someone about your worries
- Letting go
- Laughter, play, have fun
- Biofeedback techniques
- Tai Chi
- Yoga
- Focused breathing exercises
- Take a bath
- Relax with aromatherapy or candles
- Take a media break, such as no television, phone, internet, email, or social media
- Embrace silence

Let silence open up your heart so you can hear it sing.
Doreen Virtue

Being connected to nature

Being connected to nature can refresh your soul and remind you of your connectedness to the Universe. Research studies have shown that your environment can either reduce or increase your stress. Stresses in the environment can have an impact on your health and immune system.

Being in nature can help alleviate stress and increase your feelings of well-being.

Healing Gardens are green spaces, in either hospitals, hospices, or the community, that promote quiet reflection in a garden setting. Researchers in this field have found a benefit in relief from symptoms, stress reduction, sense of well-being, and hopefulness. [75]

Grounding (Earthing) – This area of emerging science has shown that walking barefoot on the Earth has a positive impact on your immune system and overall feeling of health and well-being. It is the belief that the electrons from the Earth have a healing effect on the human body. The best way to achieve this is to stand barefoot on the Earth for 10 minutes a day. There are also products that allow you to be grounded to the Earth such as sheets, blankets, and special sandals.

6 ways to communicate with nature
1. **Make a commitment to connect with nature** – Set a clear intention to connect with nature, and let it happen naturally.
2. **Create time alone in nature** – Spend time alone, as communicating with nature may work best in solitude. You could even do this in your garden or at a park.
3. **Find a good place** – Find a place that you are drawn to, and is easy to access.

4. **Sit down** – It may be easier to connect with nature if you take the time to sit down and relax.
5. **Relax and observe** – Take in the surroundings: see, hear, smell, feel, and notice the little details.
6. **Communicate** – Try to really listen and hear nature, and communicate back in your own way. Talk to the trees. [74]

I go to nature to be soothed and healed,
and have my senses put in order.
John Burroughs

Spirituality and religion

Some helpful definitions

Faith is a strong belief, either religious or spiritual, that you believe, regardless of proof.

Spirituality is a broad concept, with room for many perspectives. In general, it includes a sense of connection to something bigger than ourselves, and it typically involves a search for meaning in life.

Religion is the belief in, and worship of, a superhuman controlling power, especially a God, Goddess, or Gods.

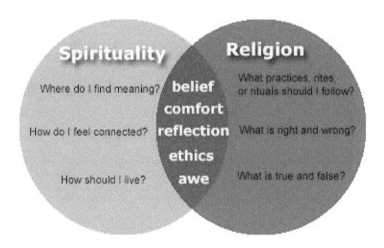

FICA approach to spiritual inquiry

The FICA questionnaire is a tool your healthcare team may use while performing a spiritual assessment.

Faith or beliefs – What do you believe in that gives meaning to your life?

Importance and influence – How important is your faith (or religion or spirituality) to you?

Community – Are you a part of a religious or spiritual community?

Address – How would you like me to address these issues in your health care?

Community support services and legacy work

We are all just humans here and we come together to share life for the day.
Barb Nolan- Day Hospice Coordinator

Day Hospice

Day hospice programs are a place where people with a life-limiting illness, along with volunteers and staff, can meet for a day of fun, relaxation, and support. Barb is a registered nurse and day hospice coordinator at Hospice Niagara. She has worked in palliative care for over 25 years and believes that hospice palliative care brings comfort and dignity to those in need, and helps to improve their quality of life. Barb affirms that "people can feel isolated at home, but through day hospice programs, they can build relationships with other people in a supportive and caring environment."

Clients are not patronized, and they are respected for what they have to offer, as everyone has something to give back. A first-day hospice participant declared, "I had such an amazing first day; I felt human again." Day hospice programs may use art and music therapies as a creative outlet. Dignity therapy and legacy work are an important part of improving quality of life for those with the illness, and helping with bereavement for those they leave behind. Bette, a day hospice participant, expressed, "You had time to talk and to listen; that's what we need, to talk about the past. I feel so much better at the end of the day."

I had the pleasure of meeting Alex, a 79-year-old gentleman, who had been diagnosed with lung cancer that had, unfortunately, spread to his body. He was not pursuing any further cancer treatments and was referred to the outpatient palliative care team for pain and symptom management, and end-of-life care. Alex and his wife, Jean, lived in a tidy little trailer in a beautiful trailer park in the country. I was met at the door by their little pet dog, Daisy. Alex was the main caregiver to his wife, Jean, after she had a stroke. His symptoms included shortness of breath and tiredness, and he was experiencing some isolation since he had become unable to drive, and Jean did not have her license. I invited Alex and Jean to join our day hospice program, and it was arranged for a volunteer to pick them both up and return them home from the day hospice. Alex, although being quite shy and reserved, found he really enjoyed the competitive card table and the lovely chef cooked meal. Jean, being very outgoing and social, enjoyed meeting people, chatting, the creative crafts activities, and after lunch entertainment. For the next several months, I continued to see both Alex and Jean in my outpatient clinic at the day hospice, or in their home at the trailer park. One day at the day hospice outpatient clinic, Alex was brought up in some distress. He had shortness of breath, was feeling very weak, and was pale and sweaty. On clinical examination, I determined that Alex, unfortunately, was actively dying from his disease. He was with

Jean who was extremely worried about him. In the past, whenever I spoke with Alex regarding his fears about death and dying, he exclaimed that "he was not worried because he was going to live to 100." When I saw Alex, I said, "I think you're dying," and he said, "I know, but I just wanted to come one more time to say goodbye." I asked him if he wanted to go home. He said no, and that he would like to stay for one more lunch and then go home. In the wheelchair, with his oxygen and his wife by his side, he did stay for one more lunch at the day hospice. He had brought with him some venison, which he had got his last time out hunting. It was his hope that Chef Patrick would be able to use it to make a meal at day hospice in the future. It was a way for him to say thank you for all that he had received. Alex was not able to eat that last meal, but he did enjoy sitting at the table, between Jean and I, quietly discussing his childhood. Jean, and some of the volunteers who knew he was dying, sat with tears in their eyes. I had made arrangements with our team nurse practitioner, Sue, and his palliative home care nurse, Dawn, to meet him at his home with end-of-life medications to start immediately. Jean called all the family to be there in his last hours. With Daisy curled up by his feet, Alex died that evening, in comfort and with dignity, surrounded by his family at home. A month later, Jean returned to day hospice, to enjoy the meal prepared by Chef Patrick, with Alex's venison. Jean continues to receive bereavement support from the team's counselors, myself, and the day hospice volunteers. She affirms that by having the whole home hospice team wrap services around Alex and herself, it had made it possible for them to cope with the challenges of end of life at home.

The following is an excerpt from a letter received from Gord, a patient with the Hospice South Niagara Palliative Outreach Team.

To Dr. Dooler and the hospice team,

I am blessed and pleased to send this letter of gratitude regarding the gift of dinner for six from M.T. Bellies family restaurant. The food, service, and your unselfish thought, was very much appreciated by us, my son, and his family. We talked about your day programs and how it helps with communication, laughter, great food, and various bands and singing, which is very therapeutic. Also, it completes a day of enjoyment with social activities with other patients and volunteers, and a visit with Dr. Dooler, or a chat with bereavement counselor, Clare.

Being a patient with Hospice South Niagara throughout the last two years has been a painful and wonderful experience, building memorable moments, making a difference, and being my authentic self. I knew my concerns and problems would be solved, as this is the best medical team we have ever been associated with; it delivers the real meaning of patient care and hope.

Hope is the lifeline of this life, and provides strength when you're alone. Just one ray of hope, when the outlook is dark, can carry you through the unknown.

Yesterday is history, tomorrow is a mystery, and today is a gift.

I wish to thank Dr. Dooler and all the team members of Hospice South Niagara for accepting me as part of your family.

Gord D.

For more information about hospice programs, or to find a hospice location near you, go to the following websites:
- National Hospice and Palliative Care Organization
- Canadian Hospice and Palliative Care Association
- Hospice Niagara

Courage is found in unlikely places.
JRR Tolkien

Visiting volunteer programs

Look for visiting volunteer programs, such as the one provided by Hospice Niagara. The visiting volunteer program provides respite for caregivers, while offering services to people with a life-limiting illness. The visiting volunteers attend a training program that teaches listening skills and how to manage grief. About 75% of the volunteers have experienced a significant loss in their life and have gravitated towards the program as a way of giving back. Volunteers are matched up with people who have common interests. They may take people shopping, to hairdressing appointments, on walks, or play games. Some volunteers will take people on outings that are interesting to them. Ann is a lovely lady with pancreatic cancer. She suffers with significant weakness and is unable to drive on her own anymore. She really enjoys meeting with her visiting volunteer, for chats and coffee. She especially enjoys going out to the casino with her. This helps her to begin to feel normal. She declares, "I love going on outings with my volunteer, especially going to the casino. This was something that I used to do before I got sick, and I am so happy that I'm able to do this now. Last time we went, I won $750 on a slot machine, and it made my day."

Legacy work

Through dignity therapy, people are given the opportunity to work on projects and leave a legacy. Projects could be written, such as a letter, poem, or book. Audio or video records can be made of their story. The value of dignity therapy comes not only with the legacy left for loved ones, but also from enjoying the process of telling the story. It gives people the opportunity to express what is important to them and can help them come to terms with their own death. It can contribute to conversations that can lead to healing.

Bereavement studies show that legacy work can help families and loved ones with their grief. One family member reminisced, "I knew the book was important to her, but now that she is gone, I really see how much it mattered."

Wellspring

Wellspring is a network of community based support centres, offering programs and services that meet the emotional, social, practical, and restorative needs of people living with cancer, and those who care for them. They offer counseling, support, mindfulness, and exercise programs for those living with cancer, and bereavement support for those left behind.

For more information, or to find a location near you, go to their website.

Other community resources

Resources in the community may include churches, synagogues, mosques, other spiritual centers, and community health centers.

Petrusia, the office assistant for the palliative care team, expresses, "It is nice to see a group of people who are available to keep people home where they are comfortable. I enjoy being part of the team and watching how people are supported." She plays an integral part of reaching out to community programs to advocate for extra resources. She affirms, "It is important for people to reach out to their community; there are often people willing to help at churches, other religious organizations, or community centers. She states, "Church resources can be utilized to help someone to clean their home, cut their grass, offer meals, and just take people for a walk." She recalls an example where many community organizations came together to grant a wish to a local family. Karen has been diagnosed with metastatic breast cancer. She lives with her husband, Kevin, and her fourteen-year-old daughter, Kristi. She was granted a wish from Dreams 2 Memories, a charitable organization that provides funding for parents with a life-limiting illness, to provide a vacation experience for their family. Her wish was to go camping at a local campground called Bissell's Hideaway. The family enjoyed their vacation wish at Bissell's. The campground generously would not accept the funding from Dreams 2 Memories and provided the holiday for free. This vacation was documented in a local newspaper. The article included a biography of Karen and her family, including their love of hockey and the rivalry between her husband, who is a Toronto Maple Leaf's fan, and her daughter, being a Montreal Canadiens fan. With the camping holiday covered by Bissell's, Dreams 2 Memories offered another opportunity. The family requested to go a Toronto versus Montreal hockey game. At the same time, the wife of a NHL referee was touched by the article in the newspaper. She contacted the palliative care team, offering to help out the family. The Leafs provided their team limousine to pick up the family to take them to the game. The NHL Referee Association provided jerseys for the family. Karen was given an official referee jersey, with her husband, Kevin, getting a Leafs jersey, and her daughter getting a Canadiens jersey. As they were sitting two rows behind the Toronto Maple Leafs bench, her daughter was given a Maple Leafs jersey by one of the players to wear, much to her dismay. The family had a night to remember.

Suggestions for things you can do to bring comfort and dignity

Tips for choosing a complementary therapy and practitioner: [70] Canadian Cancer Society
- Ask your healthcare team for help.
- Look for credible and unbiased information about the therapy.
- Evaluate the research evidence for the therapy.
- Decide what your goals are for the complementary therapy.
- Ask about the qualifications of the complementary therapy practitioner.
- Look carefully at what the therapy claims to do.
- Find out about possible side effects of the therapy.
- Find out what the complementary therapy will cost.
- Be open and honest with everyone on your healthcare team.

Visit the Canadian Cancer Society webpage for more information.

My notes, thoughts, questions, and next chapter

I highly recommend that you write down any ideas, questions, thoughts, and reflections that may be important to you. Please feel free to use your book as a companion on this, your journey, and take your book with any questions to your care providers to help start those difficult conversations.

In this chapter of *The Book on Home Hospice,* you have taken a closer look at the importance of some alternative therapies in helping to improve quality of life. You are ready now to reach the next chapter, which will discuss what to expect at the end of life. The last stages of life can be difficult and trying for you and your loved ones. An expected death at home can be an emotional roller coaster but also a rewarding and beautiful time. The next chapter will help you prepare for what is to come.

Notes

Chapter 8
What to Expect at the End of Life

Death is the wish of some, the relief of many,
and the end of all.
Lucius Annaeus Seneca (4 BC-65)
Roman philosopher and playwright

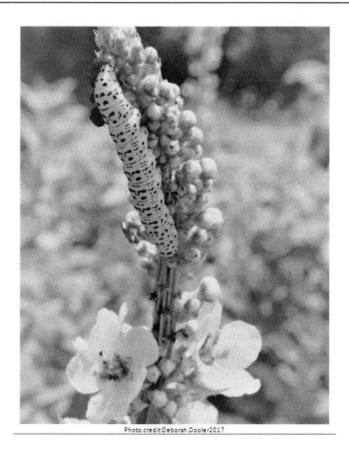

Photo.credit:Deborah.Dooler2017

Some helpful definitions

Death doula – Death midwives provide end-of-life spiritual care, rituals, and at-home funerals.

Medical assistance in dying – (CPSO) College of Physicians and Surgeons – in accordance with federal legislation, includes circumstances where a medical practitioner (i.e., physician or nurse practitioner), at an individual's request (a) administers a substance that causes an individual's death;

Or (b) prescribes or provides a substance for an individual to self-administer to cause their own death.

In the case of Carter v. Canada, the Supreme Court of Canada (SCC) unanimously determined that the Criminal Code provisions that prohibit medical assistance in dying, violate the charter rights of competent adults who are suffering intolerably from grievous and irremediable medical conditions, and who seek a physician's assistance in dying. In response, the federal government enacted legislation, through amendments to the Criminal Code, to establish a framework for medical assistance in dying in Canada. [7]

Palliative sedation – Also known as terminal sedation, it refers to the practice of relieving intolerable suffering through the proportional and monitored use of opioids and/or sedative medications to intentionally lower a patient's level of consciousness at the end of life. [7]

Continuous ambulatory delivery device (CADD pump) – A pump device for delivering continuous medication over a 24-hour period, with the ability to give yourself a bolus dose of breakthrough medication as needed, with the push of a button. It can be either intravenous (in a vein or picc line, or portacath) or sub cutaneous into the fatty tissue under the skin.

Peripherally inserted central catheter (PICC or PIC line) – Less commonly called a percutaneous indwelling central catheter, it is a form of intravenous access that can be used for a prolonged period of time (e.g., for long chemotherapy regimens, extended antibiotic therapy, or total parenteral nutrition).

Port-A-Cath – Is a small medical appliance that is installed beneath the skin. A catheter connects the port to a vein. Under the skin, the port has a septum through which drugs can be injected and blood samples can be drawn many times, usually with less discomfort for the patient than a more typical needle stick.

Organ and tissue donation – The Trillium Gift of Life Network Act – Sets out requirements relating to organ and tissue transplantation measures for health facilities designated by the Minister of Health and Long-Term Care. [7]

Autopsy – The physical examination of the body after death by a physician called a pathologist. It is usually used to precisely determine the cause of death. It is not commonly required for those who have an expected death.

Coroner – An official of a local community who holds inquests concerning sudden, violent, or unexplained deaths. It is not commonly required for those who have an expected death.

Terminal sedation versus medical assistance in dying

I met Bryan and Sue at their sprawling ranch home in the countryside, along with Sparky, the cat, and Cotton, the horse. Bryan had been diagnosed with metastatic lung cancer and had been told by his oncology team that the cancer had spread, and treatments were no longer going to be helpful. A request was made for the palliative care team to provide support and comfort at home. Bryan was originally from New Zealand, where he met his wife, a Canadian, Sue. They were married, and returned to live in Canada. Bryan was a very proud, independent, hardworking man, and he was having some difficulty adapting to the role of the sick and dying man, he felt he had become. As he became weaker and more dependent on others for his care, he began to ask about his options. He was rapidly becoming bed bound and did not want to be a burden on his family.

We discussed medical assistance in dying (MAID), which had just recently become legal in Ontario. Assisted dying is intended for capable adults whose deaths are reasonably foreseeable and who are legally eligible. [38]

I explained that medical assistance in dying involves a specialized team of professionals that will make an assessment to see if he would meet the criteria for acceptance into the program. The process has been evolving but involves two separate physician/ nurse practitioner interviews, and then a 10-day waiting period, which can be waived. If approved, the MAID team could come to the home to do the procedure, or he could go to the hospital. The procedure involves the injection of medications that would cause the heart to stop.

Medical assistance in dying (MAID) means:

The administering, by a doctor or nurse practitioner, of a substance to a person, at their request, that causes their death;

Or

The prescribing or providing, by a doctor or nurse practitioner, of a substance to a person, at their request, so that they may self-administer the substance, and in doing so, cause their own death. [38]

Medical assistance in dying is not a replacement for good quality palliative care to ease the suffering at the end of life. I explored with him his fears and concerns, and explained terminal sedation as an option.

Bryan stated that he did not want to suffer pain or anxiety, and did not want to be a burden on his family. He was not afraid to die but was afraid to suffer and cause his family suffering, watching him die.

Terminal sedation in palliative care means:

Terminal sedation is the continuous deep sedation, or sedation for intractable distress in the dying person. It is the palliative practice of relieving distress in a terminally ill person in the last hours or days of life.

And

Involves the administration of a narcotic medication on a continuous ambulatory delivery device (CADD pump), along with a sedative medication, on a continuous pump. [7]

After discussing the options, Bryan felt that he wanted to be comfortable at home. He was nearing the end of life and would not benefit from the MAID process, as his death was imminent, and he likely had less than 10 days to live. He had been able to say goodbye to his relatives who had recently visited from New Zealand, and he was ready to say goodbye to his beloved wife. I arranged for the terminal sedation pumps to be delivered, and to be started when Bryan had a chance to say, "Thank you, I love you, and farewell." His palliative nurse set up the pumps, and the medications were started with his family at the bedside. He very quickly slipped into a comfortable comatose state and died a couple of days later, quietly and peacefully, with dignity in his home, surrounded by all he loved, listening to the Eagles song, Hotel California.

The following is an excerpt from a letter that Bryan's wife, Sue, sent to his palliative team, who also looked after her dying mother:

Hi Ladies

Hope you both are well and still spreading your wonderful smiles and incredible knowledge to people in need. Words cannot express what you both did for us. I hope you got to see an obituary in the paper or at the funeral home. We have to praise you for all that you did for us. And for my Mom!!!

Actually, Sparky (the cat), Cotton (the horse), and I are doing alright. We are missing Bryan in this big quiet house now. His spirit is still with us here. Sparky has been very docile since Bryan passed, plus the fact he is missing doing your hair in the mornings!! It is hard to believe how much was going on before in our house, and then nothing....

I have to tell you what happened when they picked Bryan up to take him to the funeral home.

The two young guys came in and asked me what his favorite song was. I thought of how strange that was. I said, "Well, I had the Eagles playing first thing this morning, so probably Hotel

California." He said, "Well, we have that in the van, so we will play it all the way to the funeral home." I was speechless! He then said for all of us to go out to the veranda. He pulled up to the front of the house, rolled all the windows down, cranked up the volume, and drove so slowly all the way down our laneway. Even Cotton came over to the fence. Priceless!!

Take care for now.

Hugs
Sue

I am a person who carries a disease,
but the disease does not define all of me.
Clare Braun- Palliative Psychosocial Bereavement Counselor

Clare is a retired Baptist minister, a certified therapist, and a psychosocial bereavement counselor. He had an integral part in the formation of the outreach palliative care team. He has been a great support to me, personally, and many others on the team. He affirms, "One of the biggest things people face at the end of life is to look for meaning. They may question, "Does my life matter at all? Does my life matter to anyone?" He encourages people to find different ways to explore and seek to make meaning of these questions. Counseling either the individual or the family can be helpful. Legacy work, through day hospice or other programs, can be a very therapeutic experience for all involved. He declares, "Death has a way of sharpening the opportunity to talk about emotions in the family. The emotions that this work elicits may not be pretty, but even the darkest emotions are honest and can be healing." Clare maintains, "It is always important to remember I am a person," which are words we all can live by.

Forgiveness is a virtue of the brave.
Indira Gandhi

Dr. Ira Byock, in his book, *Dying Well: The Prospect for Growth at the End of Life,* writes about his belief that the transition to death can be one of life's most meaningful experiences. It provides an opportunity for you to grow as a person, to forgive and be forgiven, to say those things that need to be said, and hear those things that need to be heard. Communication at the end of life is important for the dying, and for those that are bereaved.

Dr. Ira Byock describes 5 things that the dying patient and family member can benefit from hearing:

1. I forgive you.
2. Forgive me.
3. Thank you.

4. I love you.
5. Goodbye. [34]

Forgiveness

People can learn and change until their last breath. You cannot alter the events of the past, but you can make a last journey back to forgive yourself and others for being imperfect rather than carry such burdens until you die. [39]

It's one of the greatest gifts you can give yourself, to forgive.
Forgive everybody.
Maya Angelou

Repentance

Many religions value repentance as a way to empty your mind of feelings of guilt, and express your regrets. It is a way of asking for forgiveness for your mortal sins. The word repentance comes from the Greek word *metanoia,* and it means turning from sin. This may be a part of your spirit beliefs or religion that is important to explore for you.

---

*Repentance means you change your mind so deeply
that it changes you.*
Bruce Wilkinson

Last few months and days

While writing this chapter on what to expect at end of life, I got a call on Saturday night from a palliative home care nurse, Laurie. She explained that John, an elderly man with metastatic prostate cancer, had a high fever with chills, sweats, restlessness, and hallucinations. John is in his last days of life and in the transitional phase of dying. With no focus of infection, the fever is likely from changes in the normal functioning of the brain to regulate body temperature. The body temperature can drastically fluctuate, causing distressing symptoms. I ordered some acetaminophen suppositories to help regulate his temperature. The next morning, Laurie contacted me to let me know that John's fever had resolved, and he was sitting up smiling and telling her the best way to cook trout. At this point, he was not able to take in anything except sips of water, but he was reminiscing about trout for breakfast and was very happy.

Laurie states, "I saw a picture on the table of John at the cottage, and I asked him about it. He told her that he would go to the cottage with his friends, and while they were all in bed sleeping, he would get up early and go fishing for trout.

Mornings are the best time to catch the fish—the earlier the better. Sometimes he would be up at 4:30 a.m., out on the water, while his friends slept. John declared, "I would go out early, catch the trout, start the camp fire, clean the fish, put the fish in foil with lots of butter, cook the fish over the fire, and then, and only then, would his friends get out of bed to the smell of the fresh-cooked fish."

I saw John the next day and, with routine acetaminophen suppositories, he was comfortable, with his family at the bedside. John is one of my patients in a retirement home, and he has a lovely grey and white cat named Sammy. Sammy has been such a good companion for John, that he could not imagine leaving his home and his precious Sammy. With Sammy cuddled on the hospital bed, I was able to say goodbye to John. He thanked me, with a very frail voice, for keeping him and Sammy home. John slipped into a coma and was transferred to Hospice Niagara, the Stabler Center, which is a residential hospice, where he died peacefully and comfortably, surrounded by his loved ones. I'm sure he was thinking about the best way to cook trout. His precious Sammy was adopted by a close family friend.

John's daughter, Shelly, a retired nurse, expressed, "I have been so overwhelmed with the support offered to my father in the retirement home, and with the palliative team services. Everyone has been wonderful, and he has had excellent care. It has allowed me and my family to take the time to say goodbye to my Dad and spend some time with him. I am very impressed with the dedication of all of the personal support workers and nurses looking after my Dad; they are so caring and kind."

Laurie declares that, "I love knowing the palliative care team is available to respond to the needs of my dying patients. With the team, you have continuity, communication, and collaboration. You can brainstorm to come up with solutions to help alleviate the suffering. Being prepared with a symptom relief kit makes a world of difference, so that I don't have to try to find help at night or on long weekends; it gives me, and my patients, peace of mind. It helps people to leave the world peacefully. We are just ever so grateful to be able to have what is needed available, and not have to wait and suffer. When somebody dies, and they are comfortable at home, surrounded by family, they are grateful. I feel privileged that we are doing what palliative care is all about."

Residential inpatient hospice

People think they are coming to hospice to die, but our goal is to help people live well until they die.
Tina Van Egmond, Hospice Niagara Director of Care

Residential hospice is a place where people with a life-limiting illness at the end of life can be cared for in a home-like environment. Most people prefer to stay in their own homes as long as possible. In some circumstances, it may not be desirable or possible to stay at home for end-of-life care. Residential hospice may be the perfect transition in this situation. Twenty-four-hour care is provided by specialized physicians, nurses, counsellors, staff, and volunteers—all people with a passion for providing palliative care.

Hospices are often more than just a building; they are integral to spreading knowledge and education regarding end-of-life care to the community, including inpatient and outpatient programs, bereavement programs, and capacity building.

Tina is a registered nurse palliative specialist, working as the Director of Care at Hospice Niagara, the Stabler Center, a residential hospice. She states, "It is an absolute privilege to be allowed into a person's life at such an intimate and personal time; it helps me to be a better person." Tina started her professional career as a labor and delivery nurse, and she explains, "That experience has helped me to be a better palliative nurse. Sadness is part of life; it is my role to support people and help them through it. Life is not perfect. It can be messy, but at hospice, we can help make it a little bit better for the dying person, as well as for their family." Tina admits that the ideal transition from home to inpatient hospice most often occurs when the admitted person has been under the care of a community palliative team. These people and their families are much calmer, and often there is less crisis management needed. They are aware of the trajectory of their disease and are more prepared for the transition into a 24-hour monitored and supported environment. Another key component of a successful transition to inpatient hospice is a physician to physician handover.

The goal of hospice palliative care is to provide the right care in the right place at the right time. Tina explains, "Sometimes people come to inpatient hospice too early. It may not be the best place for them if they are not dying. Some people do get better, and they do get discharged from hospice; this is to be celebrated."

Those who have the strength and the love to sit with a dying patient in the silence that goes beyond words will know that this moment is neither frightening nor painful, but a peaceful cessation of the functioning of the body.
Elisabeth Kubler-Ross

What to expect in the last few days and hours

Nutrition and hydration
- Reduced intake is normal at the end of life.
- Hunger and thirst make us eat and drink for survival. But we also eat out of habit, boredom, pleasure, satisfaction, or comfort, and because we choose to make it a social activity. Advanced disease can severely reduce our ability, need, or desire to eat and drink.

Withdrawal from the external world

As the end of life approaches, there is a feeling of detachment from the physical world, and a loss of interest in things formerly found pleasurable. There is a tendency to sleep more. There is less desire to talk. This is the beginning of letting go of life and preparing for death. [35]

What you can do
- Always speak gently, and identify yourself before speaking.
- Use gentle touch and provide reassurance.
- Dying requires energy and focus.
- Try not to distract the dying person from this necessary preparation.
- Allow time for silence.
- Remember that you are supporting the person to *let go*.

Symptom relief kit

Your palliative care providing team will anticipate potential complications that are common at the end of life, and have medications and strategies available to recognize and manage the associated symptoms to minimize suffering.

End of life medications and orders may include:
- Injectable narcotics for pain or shortness of breath (e.g., morphine, hydromorphone, and fentanyl).
- Injectable or sublingual sedatives for agitation and restlessness (e.g., midazolam, lorazepam).

- Injectable or oral drops for terminal secretions (e.g., scopolamine, atropine).
- Injectable antiemetic for nausea (e.g., stemetil, haloperidol).
- Injectable antipsychotic for nausea or agitation (e.g., haloperidol).
- Urinary catheter as needed (e.g., Foley in-dwelling catheter).
- Antipyretic suppositories for fever (e.g., acetaminophen suppository).
- Subcutaneous butterfly for end-of-life medications or hypodermoclysis fluid.

Transitional phase

The transitional phase of the dying process usually occurs in the last week to days of life, and may be referred to as the syndrome of imminent death. The person is actively dying, and in the final stages of the dying process you may see an increase in somnolence, weakness, decreased interest in surroundings, loss of appetite, confusion, falls, and incontinence.

Pain is reported to occur in up to 75% of dying patients, requiring opioid analgesics. A change in the route of the medication may be needed if unable to swallow. There may be shortness of breath, anorexia, or decreased oral intake.

Actively dying

In the final stages of the dying process, the body starts to slowly shut down.

Changes in skin

You may notice changes in the temperature of the skin, making it warm, or cool and clammy. As the part of the brain that controls temperature regulation shuts down, there may be fever, hypothermia, or an alternating of both. This is a normal process and not thought to be distressful; however, it may be treated with acetaminophen suppositories to relieve fever. The skin may also change color, with pale, cyanosis or blueness and mottling noted.

You may notice that the hands are cool, and the nail beds may turn dusky or blue. The mouth and skin around the mouth may also turn slightly blue or mottled.

Changes in breathing

You may notice a change in the breathing pattern. Breathing can become slower and more irregular, and there may be periods when the breathing stops, which is called apnea. Apnea generally starts for a few seconds and can last up to one minute or more. This can be very distressing to watch for family; however, it is thought not to be distressing for the person and a normal part of the dying process. There is no need to time how long the apnea lasts, and you may notice a gasping for air from time to time, but this is not an indication of distress. Commonly, there may be a Cheyne-Stokes pattern breathing, which is an abnormal pattern of breathing, characterized by progressively deeper and sometimes faster breathing, followed by a gradual decrease that results in a temporary stop in breathing, called an apnea. The pattern repeats, with each cycle usually taking 30 seconds to 2 minutes. When a person is no longer able to swallow their saliva, secretions collect in the back of the throat, called terminal secretions. The body continues to make up to 1.5 liters of saliva a day. Often referred to as the death rattle, it can occur in up to 92% of dying people. Most likely, your loved one would be unconscious at this point and not troubled with these secretions, although it can be alarming to listen to and can be treated with medications. Positioning is helpful to move the secretions. This is not thought to be distressing and does not need to be treated.

Changes in urine

As the body starts to shut down and the kidneys stop functioning, you may notice a decrease in urinary output. The urine may become dark, concentrated, and stronger smelling. Your health care team may suggest an in-dwelling Foley catheter be placed for comfort and convenience.

Changes in vital signs

Monitoring of vital signs, including blood pressure and pulse, are not necessary in a dying person; however, you may notice that the pulse gets weaker, faster, or slower, and the blood pressure gets lower.

Agitation and confusion

Terminal delirium is a near uniform experience at end of life, occurring in up to 88% of people during the final days or weeks of life. It can cause distress, both for the dying person and for the caregivers.

There may be a period where your loved one becomes agitated and delirious, with fluctuating levels of consciousness. This occurs as the brain starts to shut down and lacks oxygen. Terminal delirium can be distressing, but can be treated with sedating medications.

Changes in level of consciousness

There may be a time when your loved one is comatose or semi-comatose. It is important to remember that studies have shown that the hearing is still intact, and speaking gently to your loved one can be comforting.

Spiritual questioning

At the end of life, there may be spiritual questions and spiritual distress for your loved one. The best intervention is to acknowledge that they exist, and offer support as appropriate to their spiritual or religious beliefs.

---

*Working with the dying is like being a midwife
for this great rite of passage of death.
Just as a midwife helps a being take their first breath,
you help a being take their last breath.*
Ram Dass

---

*Free Bonus Material at my website, www.HomeHospice Book.com

Did you know?
When a person dies, their sense of hearing is the last to go.

How will I know when my loved one has died?

Final stage cessation of life

Eventually, the signs of cardiac, respiratory, and brainstem function ceases, meaning that the heart stops beating, the lungs stop breathing, and the brain activity stops.

You will notice that the skin begins to cool rapidly and become grey or dusky blue. At this time, the body may release the urine and bowel contents as the muscles in the body relax. Eventually, the muscle may become rigid or stiff; this is called rigor mortis and happens over time.

You may not have seen a dying or deceased person before, and may have worry or concerns about how you will cope at this challenging time. Studies have shown that being with a loved one at the end of life can be helpful, as you are able to comfort the dying person, express emotions, and be comforted and supported by your own family members.

It is okay to cry; it is a sad occasion. It is okay to feel relief that your loved one is no longer suffering. It is okay to feel guilt, sadness, or overwhelming grief. There is no right or wrong way to be, so just be yourself.

Tears are the silent language of grief.
Voltaire

What to do next

As the death of your loved one is expected, it is not an emergency, so you **do not call 911**. You should have a plan in place that details who to call when your loved one dies. It is usually the palliative home care nurse on call. The nurse will come out to the house to pronounce the death: this means to check for a heartbeat and breathing, and muscle stiffness, to ensure that the person has died. A physician may also come out to the house to pronounce, and sign a death certificate.

If the death is unexpected, or the circumstances involved in the death are suspicious, the police should be notified, and they may contact the local coroner to complete an investigation. An autopsy may be requested by the corner, if the death was unexpected, to determine the cause of death. In the case of palliative care and expected death, no autopsy is performed.

Physicians must ensure that caregivers are instructed regarding whom to contact when a patient is about to die, or has just died. The point of contact may vary, depending on, for example, local situations or processes, health-care teams, and whether or not the *Do Not Resuscitate Confirmation Form* is completed. [7]

Death certificate

A physician will need to sign a death certificate to accompany the body to the funeral home; this can usually be completed within 24 hours.

Organ and tissue donation

It is important to fully discuss your wishes regarding tissue or organ donation upon your death, before your death. This can be done by signing your driver's license to agree to organ donation, signing a donation card, putting your wishes in your will, discussing your wishes for organ donation with your family and health care providers, or online.

The Government of Canada supports organ and tissue donation and transplantation. The provinces and territories are responsible for maintaining the program in their jurisdiction. In Ontario, contact Trillium Gift of Life, at BeADonor.ca.

Visit your government website for more information.

Caution
Do not post notice of the death on any social media sites, such as Facebook, Instagram, Twitter, and Snapchat, until all family and friends have been notified in person.

*Free Bonus Material at my website, www.HomeHospice Book.com

Who to contact

- Contact your healthcare provider first to come to the house to pronounce the death and arrange for the completion of a death certificate.
- Contact your local funeral home to make arrangements to pick up your loved one's body. You may need a burial permit in your jurisdiction.
- Contact your family and friends who need to be notified of the death.
- Contact your local organ donation program if that was your loved one's wishes.

- Reach out to your religious or spiritual community to inform them of the death, and request support.
- Notify your loved one's employer, if applicable.
- Stop income sources, such as pensions (CPP, ONA), Hoop, WSIB, Veterans Affairs, disability insurance.
- Contact Canada Pension and Old Age Security for applications for lump-sum death benefit, Survivor, or Children's Benefits.
- Contact the insurance companies to inform them of the death and request information regarding how to file a claim.
- Contact your lawyer to determine if there is a will and who is executor.
- Contact home help, nursing services, and meals on wheels to cancel services.

Documents to Gather

- Social Insurance Number
- Birth Certificate
- Health Card
- Marriage Certificate
- Voided cheque for CPP survivors benefit
- Copy of power of attorney
- Current tax return of deceased, and T-slips
- Life Insurance documents
- Copy of Last Will and Testament

Bustle in the House
The Morning after Death
Is solemnest of Industries
Enacted upon Earth
Emily Dickenson

My notes, thoughts, questions, and next chapter

I highly recommend that you write down any ideas, questions, thoughts, and reflections that may be important to you. Please feel free to use your book as a companion on this, your journey, and take your book with questions to your care providers to help start those difficult conversations.

In this chapter of *The Book on Home Hospice,* you have learned what the end days may look like and what to expect. In the next chapter of *The Book of Home Hospice,* you will learn what comes next after the death of your loved one, including who to call, funeral and memorial services, donation of organs and tissue, and whole-body donation, and your legal obligations.

Notes

_____

_____

_____

_____

_____

_____

_____

_____

_____

_____

_____

_____

_____

_____

_____

_____

_____

_____

_____

_____

_____

_____

_____

_____

_____

Notes

Chapter 9
What Comes After Death

The life of the dead is placed in the memory of the living.
Marcus Tullius Cicero

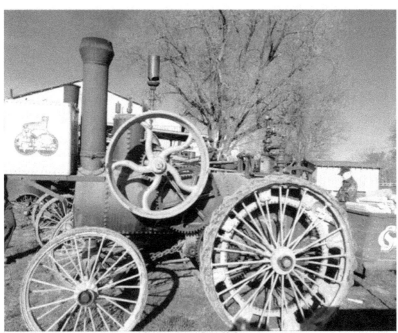
Photo.credit:John.Dooler2015

Did you know?
In 1845, United States' President Andrew Jackson's pet parrot was removed from his funeral for swearing.

Some helpful definitions:

Body donation – your whole body is donated to a medical school, or school of anatomy, for educational and research purposes only. Remains are respectfully cremated and are interred in the school's plot, or they may be returned to the family upon request. It is important that you make your wishes, to donate your body, known to your next-of-kin. You may also indicate your wishes in your will. [43]

Celebration of life – a memorial, or a fabulous farewell; these gatherings are typically held apart from a funeral or religious ceremony.

Cremation – the processing of a dead person's body by burning it to ashes; this can be done before or after a ceremony.

Crypt – an underground room or vault beneath a church, used as a chapel or burial place.

Digital legacy – includes everything digital that you leave behind upon your death, including computer hardware, software, and your online presence.

Earth burial – the internment of a body in a casket, or the cremated remains into a grave.

Entombment – the placing of a dead body in a tomb, mausoleum, or crypt.

Eulogy – a speech or writing in praise of a person(s) or thing(s), especially one who recently died or retired, or as a term of endearment. Eulogies may be given as part of funeral services. They may take place in a funeral home during or after a wake. [41]

Funeral – a ceremony connected with the burial or cremation of the body of a dead person, or the burial (or equivalent) with the attendant observances. [41] A funeral service is a service held to memorialize a deceased person, with their body present. [42]

Mausoleum – a building, especially a large and stately one, housing a tomb or tombs.

Memorial Service – a service held to memorialize a deceased person, with their body not present, or cremated remains present. [42]

Obituary – a news article that reports the recent death of a person, typically along with an account of the person's life, and information about the upcoming funeral. [41] It can be in a paper or on the internet.

Organ or tissue donation – the donation of organs or tissue to a living person.

Ritual – a sequence of activities involving gestures, words, and objects, performed in a sequestered place, and performed according to set sequence. Rituals may be prescribed by the traditions of a community, including a religious community. [41]

Visitation – a time for mourners to view the body (may have an open or closed casket). [40]

Wake – a social gathering associated with death, usually held before a funeral. Traditionally, a wake takes place in the house of the deceased. [41]

Caution
Do not post notice of the death on any social media sites, such as Facebook, Instagram, Twitter, and Snapchat, until all family and friends have been notified in person.

Contacting family and friends

Did you know?
The creator of the Pringles packaging had his ashes stored in a Pringles can after he died.

After your loved one has died, it is very important to allow enough time to contact all family members personally to let them know of the death. This includes monitoring that the death is not announced on social media sites, such as Facebook, Instagram, Twitter, or Snapchat, before all family and friends have been notified. It can be traumatic for family to find out about the loss on social media before being told in person. This becomes more and more important as tweeting and posting statuses becomes an instant way of communicating.

What information to give regarding funeral or memorial services:
- The date of the service.
- The location of the service.
- The time that the service will be held.
- Details about pre-service or post-service events.
- If you are accepting donations to charity in the name of the person who died.
- Where flowers can be sent, or if you would prefer not to receive flowers.

Minors and dependant adults

If there are minor children or other dependent adults, the priority is their safety. Arranging for temporary care for any minor children, or other dependents of the deceased, should be your priority. You may initially need to consider daycare, or temporarily asking for assistance from your family and friends. It is important to remember that this is a difficult time for everyone involved. Children and dependent adults can be especially vulnerable at this time. In addition to concerns regarding their physical safety, consideration should be given to emotional support and counseling.

Minor children

In the case of minor children, the remaining parent will be considered the guardian. A guardian is a person granted physical custody of the child and who is responsible for their care until they reach the age of eighteen. In a Will, the parent may nominate a guardian, if both parents are deceased. A guardian can only be established by the Courts, although, most likely, they may consider the parents' wishes. The Court may appoint a different guardian if it is in the child's best interest. If both parents are deceased, and the child inherits assets from the estate, a Trustee may have been appointed in the parents' Will. This person will manage the assets of the child until they are age eighteen, or otherwise as arranged in the trusteeship.

Dependent adults

Dependent adults being cared for by the deceased will need to be cared for and supported at this difficult time. It is important to determine whether the dependent adult has a power of attorney or living trust established. If so, this person should be advised of the death of the caregiver. If no previous trust has been determined, then the Court may establish a conservatorship for the adult. A conservatorship allows the conservator to have authority over both physical care and financial matters. [77]

To obtain for more information regarding guardianship or conservatorship, please contact your lawyer.

Dealing with social media and online accounts

Digital legacy

A digital legacy includes everything digital that you leave behind upon your death, including computer hardware, software, and your online presence. In the past twenty years, the cyber world has become a large part of our lives. We have seen a transition to a mostly online and paperless society. This change will have an impact upon how information is accessed and managed by loved ones after your death. You may have photos, videos, cyber assets, and information that you would like to pass on to future generations. At the same time, there may be information online that you do not want accessed. Digital photos, videos, or love letters in the form of emails or texts, may have as much sentimental value as those in the physical world.

Consider who should have access to your social media, photos, videos, emails, file storage, video games, and personal or business websites. Taking steps to manage your virtual life, and determine who has access to various accounts, can be as important as writing a Will for your property and physical assets. As part of estate planning, you should consider what will happen to online accounts, blogs, social media, and digital files when you die.

The first step is becoming aware of your digital presence and keeping good records. Document the user name, password, and answers to secret questions, along with who you want to access each online account.

For more information on leaving a digital legacy, please visit my website at **www.HomehospiceBook.com.**

Online companies can provide a digital safety box where you can store all your account information in one place, with a beneficiary listed for each account. It is important to remember that online companies come and go, and you will need to ensure that your data and privacy will remain safe. Check with your local authorities regarding digital property asset laws.

If no prior arrangements have been made for online accounts, they will remain active unless someone contacts the website to let them know of your death, or the account is not used for a specified amount of time. Upon death, accounts are non-transferable and will be deleted or deactivated. Your family can request the accounts be deactivated by providing appropriate identification and copy of a death certificate. Family members or executors may request a court order to access the information in your accounts, which may be granted depending on the laws of your local authority or the laws of the location of the online account, which may be in another country. Canceling your accounts can protect from identity theft and fraud.

Social networks: Facebook, Instagram, LinkedIn, Twitter, Pinterest, dating sites, etc.

Each company has its own policies regarding accessing online accounts after death.

Blogs and licensed domain names: If you are a blogger, consider having your executor take down the blog and let your readers know about your death. Blogging can be financially rewarding in the form of sponsored banner ads. The executor needs to know how to address this. If you own a domain name, consider what you wish to happen to it on your death.

Photos, music, and files: The Cloud, Dropbox, YouTube, Spotify, iPlayer, Kindle, Kobo, Flickr, Picasa, etc.

You can leave instructions on how to access these accounts, with your executor. If no instructions are left, eventually the account will be disabled and inaccessible. Online music and books may not be transferable once you die, unlike a regular book or CD.

Sellers and buyers accounts: Amazon, eBay, Etsy, etc.

Leave instructions for your executor regarding what to do with your store, if you are a seller. It may be important for someone to have access to your accounts, as there may be outstanding business for your estate to deal with.

Online streaming accounts: Netflix, Hulu, Amazon Prime, Apple TV, Crave, etc.

Contact the online providers to let them know of the death, as there may be ongoing charges to the account.

Online currencies: Linden dollar, Bitcoin, World of Warcraft currency, PayPal, Air miles, Aeroplan miles, etc.

Online currencies may be considered an asset to your estate, and your executor should have information on how to access them.

Other online accounts: gaming, gambling, online poker, PlayStation, Xbox, MLB.com, NFL.com, Satellite radio.

Online gaming and gambling is a huge multimillion dollar business. There may be assets in these accounts that can be transferred to beneficiaries.

Managing email accounts

Email providers: Yahoo, Google (Gmail), Microsoft (Hotmail), AOL, employer email, etc.

Each email provider may have a different policy regarding death. The account may be deleted, depending on the company's policy. You can direct your executor to access your account by giving your passwords before they are deactivated.

Religious or spiritual organizations

Reach out to your religious or spiritual organizations and ask to speak to your pastor, rabbi, priest, or other clergy. Notify them of the death and request their involvement in funeral or memorial services, if that was your loved one's wishes. They may offer to come to the home to be a supportive presence while you contact family and friends at this difficult time.

Funeral arrangements

A funeral is a ceremony connected with the burial or cremation of a body of a dead person. A funeral service is held to memorialize a deceased person with their body present, and a memorial service is held to memorialize a deceased person with the body not present. A funeral may have a visitation time for mourners to view the body with an open or closed casket. There may be rituals associated with a funeral prescribed by the traditions of the community or religious community. Along with the trend towards a home death, there is also a trend towards rituals and ceremonies performed in the home instead of a funeral parlor. This is a trend that has come full circle, back to the early part of the 20th century, when a loved one's body was viewed and memorialized in the home. As funeral services and burial have been becoming more expensive, there have been more options for alternative funeral arrangements at a lower price point. Celebration of life services have become more popular in the past decade. A celebration of life service is a memorial, or fabulous farewell, that brings together people to celebrate the life of the deceased person. Due to financial or personal beliefs, more and more people are choosing to have no ceremony on their death. There is no right and wrong way to memorialize the passing of a loved one. It can be important to have discussions with your family members about what your wishes are, and how you wish to be remembered. Funeral pre-planning is a good idea and can alleviate added stress for family members after your death. Some options include cremation, which is the burning of the deceased body, or burial in a casket. Another option that you may consider is the donation of your body for medical research; this can be arranged through your local anatomical board. Body donation means that your whole body is donated to a medical school, or school of anatomy, for educational and research purposes only. Remains are respectfully cremated and are interred in the school's plot, or they may be returned to the family upon request. It is important that you make your wishes, to donate your body, known to your next-of-kin. You may also indicate your wishes in your will. Tissue or organ donation does not generally interfere with funeral arrangements.

Alan D. Wolfelt, in his book, *Creating Meaningful Funeral Ceremonies: A Guide for Caregivers,* suggests that meaningful funeral ceremonies can and do make a significant difference in how the bereaved channel their grief toward health and healing.

Meaningful funerals are doorways to healing for the bereaved.

Purpose of the meaningful funeral:
- Confirm that someone we loved has died.
- Help us understand that death is final.
- Allow us to say goodbye.
- Serve as a private and public transition between our lives before the death to our lives after death.
- Encourage us to embrace and express our pain.
- Help us remember the person who died and encourage us to share those memories with others.
- Offer a time and place for us to talk about the life and death of the deceased.
- Affirm the worth of our relationship with the person who died.
- Provide a social support system for us and other mourners.
- Help integrate mourners back into the community.
- Allow us to search for meaning in life and death.
- Reinforce the fact of death in all our lives.
- Establish ongoing helping relationships among mourners. [40]

Legal and financial obligations

Death registration

The funeral director will help with this process: two documents must be submitted to the municipal clerk's office in your jurisdiction.

Medical Certificate of Death is completed by the most responsible physician.

Statement of Death is to be completed by a family member and a funeral director, and provides personal information about the deceased. [44]

Employer

You will need to notify your loved one's employer immediately after the death. At this time, you should request information regarding last payments, survivor benefits, insurance policies, and who is designated as beneficiary. You may need to arrange to have their belongings gathered from the workplace for pickup.

Lawyer regarding will and estate

Contact your loved one's lawyer regarding any outstanding wills and estate planning, and to determine who the executor of the estate is. A will is a legal document that sets out who will inherit property, possessions, and other personal items. To find out if a will has been filed, you can contact the estates division of the local court in the community where the deceased lived. Without a will, an estate is distributed according to the law. This can be a complex process. If you are in this situation, you might want to contact a lawyer. To find a lawyer, The Law Society of Upper Canada offers a free referral service by phone. [44]

Estate executor

If the executor is someone other than yourself, you should contact the designated executor of the estate to inform them of the death.

Insurance companies

Contact all the insurance companies involved to inform them of the death, and request information regarding how to file a claim. You will need to submit a death certificate and establish proof of claim. The following are some generalized steps to complete a life insurance claim.

- Obtain the policy or policy certificate number if possible.
- Determine if it's an individual policy or if it's a group/association/work policy, and who to contact to make the claim.
- Obtain the necessary forms from the broker or insurance company, complete, and return to them.
- Complete claims form.
- Provide certificate of death. A copy of the death certificate can be obtained from the funeral home. There may be a nominal fee for this.
- Provide completed doctor's report. The most responsible physician looking after your loved one should be provided with the doctor's form to fill out. There may be a fee associated with this.
- Return the completed claims form, certificate of death, and doctor's form to the insurance company. [45]

Financial institutions

It should be determined who the executor of the deceased estate is. The executor of the estate should then contact institutions to notify them of the death.

Government agencies

The estate executor is responsible for cancelling a driver's license and requesting a refund, for contacting any government agency, such as workman's compensation board, pensions, and benefits, for contacting Service Canada for health card cancellation, and for contacting any government agencies, such as family responsibilities office. Property taxes and utilities should be transferred or cancelled at the appropriate municipal level. [44]

Taxation agency (Revenue Canada)

The executor is responsible for filing an income tax return on behalf the deceased person. You can be referred to an accountant through one of three professional associations:

- Chartered Accountants of Canada
- Institute of Chartered Accountants of Ontario
- Certified General Accountants Association of Ontario

Firearms and restricted and prohibited weapons

The executor of the estate is responsible for the legal possession, or transfer and transport of, firearms and restricted or prohibitive weapons. In Canada, the Royal Canadian Mounted Police, under the firearms act, has the latest information upon the legalities of this. Check with your local authorities as to your legal responsibilities in your area. [46] Even if an individual is not personally licensed to possess firearms, they can possess a firearm left in an estate for a reasonable amount of time while the estate is being settled. An individual who is under a court-ordered prohibition from possessing firearms cannot take possession of firearms left in an estate. They can, however, act as executor and facilitate the transfer of the firearm(s) to someone who may lawfully acquire them.

Cancellation of credit cards, cell phones, and memberships

Cancelling any credit cards after death is important to help prevent identity theft or fraud. There may be automatically renewing accounts on the credit card that you do not wish to continue. Any money that is owed on a credit card should be paid before the card is cancelled.

Cellular phone contracts should be transferred or cancelled; there should not be a fee charged for this. Cell phone companies may acquire a copy of the death certificate to cancel the account. Any paid memberships should be cancelled, including gym and sports clubs. Newspaper and magazine subscriptions, both paper and virtual, will need to be canceled.

*Free Bonus Material at my website, www.HomeHospice Book.com

My notes, thoughts, questions, and next chapter

I highly recommend that you write down any ideas, questions, thoughts, and reflections that may be important to you. Please feel free to use your book as a companion on this, your journey, and take your book with your questions to your care providers to help start those difficult conversations.

In this chapter of *The Book on Home Hospice,* you have gained some knowledge about what comes next after death. In the next chapter, you will begin to understand grief, bereavement, and the stages of mourning.

Notes

_____

_____

_____

_____

_____

_____

_____

_____

_____

_____

_____

_____

_____

_____

_____

_____

_____

_____

_____

_____

_____

_____

_____

_____

Notes

_____

_____

_____

_____

_____

_____

_____

_____

_____

_____

_____

_____

_____

_____

_____

_____

_____

_____

_____

_____

_____

_____

_____

_____

Chapter 10
Life After Death – Moving On

We hug
We laugh
We cry
We love
Elizabeth J Latimer

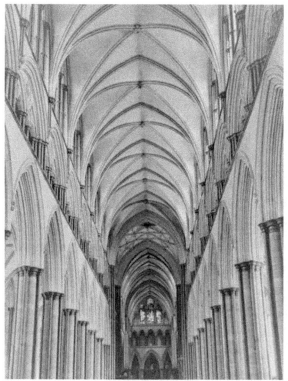

Photo.credit:Deborah.Dooler2017

Some helpful definitions:

Attachment Theory – John Bowlby is a British psychiatrist. His theory of attachment and loss suggest humans make strong affectionate bonds with others for the purpose of survival. The stronger the bond, the greater effect of the loss.

Bereavement – refers to the state, or fact, of having lost a loved one by death.

Grief – a multifaceted response to loss, particularly to the loss of someone or something that has died. [41] Grief describes the intense emotions one experiences following a loss.

Loss – the state, or feeling of grief, when deprived of someone or something of value. This could be the loss of a loved one, a divorce, the end of an intimate relationship, loss of a job, pet, or some other loss.

Mourning – in the simplest sense, is grief over someone's death. The word is also used to describe a cultural complex of behaviours in which the bereaved participate or are expected to participate. Customs vary between cultures and evolve over time, though many core behaviors remain constant. [41]

Thanatology – the scientific study of death and the practices associated with it, including the study of the needs of the terminally ill and their families. Themes include terminal illness and bereavement.

The 5 Stages of Grief – a framework for understanding and working through grief, developed by Elisabeth Kubler-Ross and David Kessler in their book titled, *Grief and Grieving: Finding the Meaning of Grace Through Five Stages of Loss*. The stages are denial, anger, bargaining, depression, and acceptance. Not everyone goes through all the stages, or in any particular order.

The biological theory of grief – There is evidence that all humans, across all cultures, past and present, grieve a loss. Grieving is seen in the animal world, with dolphins showing evidence of grief and depression after losing a mate, by refusing to eat and play. There are biological and adaptive reasons for the grieving process that are instinctive and protective after a loss. For example, the shock, numbness, and lack of feelings experienced early in the grieving process provides a protective response, which allows you to carry on with difficult tasks ahead of you, and protect you against the intense pain that you may otherwise feel.

The three R's of grief – The three common reactions to death of a loved one are:

- Realize that the person has died and realize the pain of the loss.
- Recognize the significance of the loss for you and your life.
- Rebuild your life without your loved one. [47]

The three phases of grief – According to Dr. Theresa Rando, the three phases of grief reaction are the avoidance phase, the confrontation phase, and the establishment or accommodation phase.

The avoidance phase – You begin to acknowledge and understand the death, by recognizing the loss.

The confrontation phase – You react to the separation experience and react to the losses. You may relive, review, and remember your loved one. You will begin to relinquish all the attachments and old assumptions of the world.

The accommodation phase – involves readjusting to the new world, putting your energy into new people and new goals for yourself.

Stages of recovery – These are a necessary and natural part of the healing process. As a recovery happens, it can be important to trust the process and surrender to it. The stages of recovery vary in intensity and duration, and are unique to each person and with each loss. The effects of loss can be cumulative, and one loss may bring up unresolved grief from losses in the past. [48]

Shock/ denial/numbness – These are your body's natural protective mechanisms against the intense pain that can be felt immediately and early in the process. Your mind may protect you from pain by denying the loss; you may say, "I cannot believe it is true."

Fear/anger/depression – You may expect to feel afraid of what the future will bring to you. You may be afraid of your own death or the death of others around you. You may be afraid that you will not be able to cope; you may fear being alone. Another common fear is the fear of being rejected and never being loved or being able to love again. Anger is common; it is okay to be angry. It will eventually pass. People are often angry with their loved ones, with themselves, with the medical community, or with God. There may be feelings of guilt. Depression is a deep sadness that you may feel with the loss of a loved one. It's okay to feel depressed or low for a while as you adjust. Crying can be very helpful; it can be cleansing and purifying.

Understanding/acceptance/moving on – With time and recovery, and as your mind and body are healing, you begin to understand and accept the loss. You will begin to come to a point where you realize that you can continue your life without your loved one in it. [48]

Worden's 4 tasks of grieving – a model of the process of mourning with tasks that must be accomplished, to help you come to terms with the loss and learn how to integrate it into your life. It's a flexible model where you can move backwards and forwards through the tasks in your own time. [54]

To accept the reality of the loss – This may take time and involves intellectual and emotional acceptance.

Work through the pain and grief – requires working through your emotions and feelings.

Adjust to the environment in which the deceased is missing – going back to school or work.

External adjustments – in the environment of your life.

Internal adjustments – in the way you think and feel about your life.

Spiritual adjustments – in the way you think and feel about your spiritual beliefs and religion.

To emotionally relocate the deceased and move on with life – allowing you to continue living and get on with your life.

Bereavement, grief, and mourning

Mourning is, in the simplest sense, grief over someone's death. The word is also used to describe a cultural complex set of behaviours in which the bereaved are expected to participate. Customs and rituals vary between cultures and evolve over time, though many core behaviors remain constant. [41] Although traditional mourning customs almost always involve a timeline, time doesn't heal—only grieving heals. [55] To accept the reality of the loss, involves intellectual and emotional acceptance [54]. When an emotional injury takes place, such as the death of a loved one, you begin a process of healing, as natural as the healing of a physical wound [48]. Just as a physical injury goes through a predictable cascade of steps toward healing, there are a number of tasks of mourning that lead to recovery. The tasks of mourning include the acceptance of the reality of the loss. This may take time as you work through the pain of the grief. You must adjust to living in an environment in which your deceased loved one is missing. That includes making external adjustments, internal adjustments, and spiritual adjustments, allowing you to get on with your life.

Common grief reactions – can be categorized into four areas: feelings and emotions; physical complaints; cognitive (mind) changes; and behaviours.

Feelings and emotions

Sadness – The most common feeling to experience after losing a loved one is sadness. This may or may not include crying. Studies have revealed that not allowing sadness to be expressed can lead to complicated bereavement.

Anger – Is frequently felt after a loved one has died. You may be angry for the dying person leaving you. Anger often comes from a sense of frustration; it may also stem from the fear, panic, and anxiety of being left alone and helpless. Anger can be misdirected towards those that you may blame for the death, including healthcare workers, family, God, or yourself. If anger is not acknowledged, it can lead to complicated bereavement.

Guilt – A common theme that can be related to the deceased or the circumstances of the death. It can stem from feelings of having not been able to do enough, not getting medical attention soon enough, etc. There may be guilt around things that were said or not said. There may be guilt around not being with the loved one at the end when they died. The guilt you feel most likely may be irrational; however, there may be real reasons for your guilt, and it should be explored, or this can lead to complicated bereavement.

Anxiety – Can stem from feelings of insecurity and panic. You may be worried about not being able to take care of yourself or others. There can also be anxiety and worry regarding your own mortality, as there can be a heightened sense of awareness of your own impending death.

Fears – Sleep may be affected due to a fear of dreaming, a fear of being alone, or a fear of not waking. You may have a fear of your own death, with a heightened sense of mortality.

Loneliness – Is felt by many people. It could be an emotional loneliness due to missing your loved one, or a social loneliness due to isolation.

Fatigue – A subjective feeling of tiredness, and it may have physical, mental, or emotional causes. It can often lead to apathy and listlessness.

Helplessness – Can be closely related to the fear and anxiety of feeling that you cannot care for yourself. You may feel deprived of strength and be incapacitated at times.

Shock – Most often occurs after a sudden death but can occur even after an expected death. It is usually an early emotion and a protective mechanism.

Numbness – The lack of feelings, usually felt early in the death process, and a normal protective response. It may be associated with being shocked and stunned at the death.

Suicidal ideation – Thoughts of suicide are common in the grieving process. They are often fleeting, and resolve on their own, and can be a natural symptom of pain. If you have thoughts of suicide, it is important to talk to somebody and let somebody know. If you have a plan for suicide, or feel out of control, that is a medical emergency, and you should call 911 or your local suicide prevention hotline.

Yearning – Also known as pining, is a feeling of intense longing, craving, or desire for that which is lost. It is a normal response and usually clears over time. Extended yearning is a sign of complicated bereavement.

Emancipation – The release from the care, responsibility, and control of one's parents or spouse. It can be a positive feeling after the death of an overbearing parent or spouse. It may be uncomfortable at first, and can be associated with feelings of guilt.

Relief – There are many reasons for feeling relief on the death of a loved one. You may have relief that they are no longer suffering or in pain, or you may feel relief from the release of an oppressive or abusive relationship.

Acceptance – This may not be a happy phase, and may feel more like a lack of emotion or neutral time, void of feelings. [54] [48]

It is during our darkest moments
that we must focus to see the light.
Aristotle

Physical complaints

Heart palpitations and heart pain – a sensation of heaviness in the chest and a racing heartbeat. *Broken heart syndrome* can manifest as physical changes due to a significant emotional or physical stress. Chest pain, heart palpitations, heaviness, and pressure in the chest can be signs of a heart attack. You should seek medical assistance and call 911.

Dizziness – The sensation of feeling faint, woozy, weak, or unsteady.

Trembling or tremor – Shaking or quivering of the body. Usually due to shock or excitement.

Aches and pains – Headaches, muscle aches, back, neck, and rib aches, and chest pain.

Shortness of breath – You may have difficulty breathing.

Digestive upset – Appetite loss, overeating or under eating, nausea, indigestion, constipation or diarrhea, weight loss or weight gain.

Sleep disturbances – Insomnia (not being able to fall asleep, stay asleep, or early waking), sleeping too much, vivid dreams. This will usually correct itself; however, you may need to see your physician for a medication. If sleep disorder persists, it may be a sign of depression and needs to be evaluated. It may be associated with a fear of dreaming, a fear of being alone, or a fear of not waking.

Sexual drive – Your sexual desire can be closely affected by your emotions. You may have lost your romantic partner. There may be a temporary loss of sexual functioning. You may have a lower sex drive or a higher sex drive.

Lowered immune function – Can lead to infections, and lack of energy and fatigue.

Extreme physical tiredness – Low energy and lack of motivation.

Denial helps us to pace our feelings of grief.
There is a grace in denial.
It is nature's way of letting in only as much as we can handle.
Elisabeth Kubler-Ross

Cognitive changes and behaviours

Denial and disbelief – Are thought patterns that can be protective, and allow for time to adjust to the loss.

Confusion – Your thoughts may be disorganized; you may have difficulty concentrating and become forgetful; for example, losing your car keys. In the grieving process, you may find it difficult to concentrate; you feel you cannot think straight. You may find it difficult to make decisions.

Preoccupation – Obsessive thoughts of the deceased, or excessive images of the deceased.

A sense of the deceased's presence – There may be times when you think the deceased person is still with you. In a study of bereaved children, 81% of the children stated they could sense their dead parent.

Hallucinations – Visual or auditory hallucinations may be occurring, and are especially prevalent in people with a strong spiritual or mystical belief system.

Social withdrawal – Can be caused by a tendency to withdraw into yourself emotionally. Or a physical withdrawal from the social activities you used to do.

Dreams of the deceased – You may have vivid dreams of your deceased loved one, which may be comforting or distressing.

Crying – The death of someone you love is an emotional experience, and crying is a normal reaction to this. Although crying is not necessary, and some people may not cry, it does not mean that they are not grieving.

Taking on the traits of the deceased – You may appear to develop the traits of the deceased individual, and you may wear their clothes or pick up their habits.

Inability to function – You may have difficulty coping and functioning with your life.

Restlessness, agitation, or hostility – Are behaviors that are common after a loss.

Causes for concern

Overworking – Working excessively to avoid the pain of the loss can cause an increased risk to your health due to stress.

Increased alcohol or drug intake – Using substances as a way to deal with pain and to escape grieving can lead to complicated grief and addiction issues.

Unnatural attachment to objects – Becoming irrationally attached to an object that belonged to the deceased, such as clothing and furniture, can be a sign of complicated grief.

Thoughts of suicide – Feeling out of control, like your life has lost meaning, and having a plan to complete suicide. [47]

Are you having thoughts of suicide?
Do you have a plan?
Have you attempted suicide in the past?
Do you feel out of control?

If you answered yes to any one of the above questions, please seek help now.
Tell someone you trust.
Call your family physician or bereavement support team.
If this is an emergency, call 911 or your local suicide prevention hotline.
Remember You Are Not Alone

Complicated grief

Complicated, unresolved grief is more common in people with on-going mental health issues, such as anxiety, depression, and psychotic disorders. It is more common with conjugal bereavement, which is the loss of a spouse. After the death of a spouse, you are more likely to suffer more depression in the first year. [54] Those people identified as having risk factors for complicated bereavement should be referred to a bereavement service for counseling.

The Brat Manual risk indicators for complicated bereavement

- Kinship – Was there a death of a spouse or a parent?
- Caregiver – Were you in the role of the primary caregiver to the deceased?
- Previous mental health diagnosis – such as stress, depression, and psychiatric disorders, including schizophrenia, phobias, personality disorders, and cognitive impairment, including stroke, traumatic brain injury, and dementia.
- Poor coping history – including substance abuse and suicidal history.
- A lack of spirituality or religion.
- Concurrent stressors, including caregiving of a parent or handicapped child, insufficient financial resources, other non-death losses, life-threatening illness, and previous bereavement.
- A lack of social supports.

Protective factors against complicated bereavement

- Belief in your own ability to cope.
- Strong, solid support system.
- An attitude of optimism.
- Spiritual or religious coping. [51]

When to call for help:
- If you are feeling suicidal, call 911 or your local suicide prevention hotline.
- If you are having chest pain, heart palpitations, or heaviness and pressure in the chest, this can be signs of a heart attack. You should seek medical assistance and call 911.
- If you are feeling like you are losing control.
- If you have a history of emotional disturbance.
- If you are turning to alcohol, drugs, or other addictions.
- If you feel isolated.

He who has no time to mourn has no time to mend.
John Donne

Sandra is a social worker on the palliative outreach team, and works as a psychosocial, bereavement counselor. She shares some strategies that she was used after the death of her own mother. She affirms, "Sometimes things become more significant after the death of a loved one, and things become more relevant. After my mom died, I would find messages that were very meaningful to me, and I found comfort in that. I was given a journal by some thoughtful colleagues, and I have found it a way to talk to my mother in private, as if she were still here. I take it everywhere with me, and when I want to talk to her, I write it down." Journaling can be a way to express your feelings and emotions in a safe and private way. Sandra maintains, "You can journal any unrealized goals or dreams. It can allow you to grieve your lost future." Another way to express your feelings and to ask for forgiveness, or just say what you can't say in person, is to write a letter. You can write what you would like to say to the person, as if he or she were there in front of you. You can choose to send the letter, to keep it, or to discard it. It can be a very liberating way to help with forgiving yourself and finding some peace, whether or not the other person wants to reconcile and forgive you.

You Are Not Alone

Loss is a part of life, and death is a part of life. Everyone experiences loss. You can expect you are going to have ups and downs, and good times and bad times. Grief, like love, is immeasurable. Studies show that people who take care of themselves are more able to avoid burnout. Make sure you breathe, rest, eat a healthy diet, stick to your schedule, and keep decision-making to a minimum in the immediate time frame after the death. Your feelings are unique and personal to you. Remember that feelings have no moral value; they are not good or bad–they simply exist. It's okay to feel sad and lonely; it's also okay to feel happy and laugh. Be grateful for the simple things you have in your life. There is always something to be thankful for: like a sunny day, a good cup of coffee, a family member's embrace, and a warm bed. Take each day as it comes, and try to find the hidden blessings in life.

Some days are better, some days are worse.
Look for the blessing instead of the curse.
Be positive, stay strong, and get enough rest.
You can't do it all, but you can do your best.
Unknown Author

Find ways to release your emotions:
- Beat a pillow
- Cry
- Scream
- Stomp
- Yell

Use mindfulness techniques:
- Be grateful and give thanks for all the good left in your life.
- Look for the silver lining in every situation.
- Visualizations
- Meditation
- Breathing exercises
- Laughter
- Humor
- Exercise, including tai chi and yoga
- Go for a walk
- Be in nature
- Pray
- Listen to music

- Seek out opportunities to talk:
- Talk to your doctor or nurse.
- Talk to someone at your church, synagogue, mosque, or other place of religion.
- Attend a bereavement support group.
- Talk with friends.
- Seek counseling.

Find ways to express yourself:
- Writing and journaling, to express yourself and your emotions and feelings on paper.
- Arts, hobbies, and crafts
- Singing and dancing can be therapeutic.

Find ways to say goodbye:
- Writing a letter to your deceased loved one.
- Use prayer as a way of saying goodbye.
- Visit your loved one's grave or memorial site.

Life, Love, Memories
John Dooler

Examples of Grief Rituals
- Buy a very special candle and light it at times that are special to your loved one's memory (e.g., birthday, Father's Day, anniversaries, etc.).

- Write special notes in balloons and let them go.
- Feed the hungry/homeless at Thanksgiving, holidays, etc., in memory of the loved one.
- Create a scrapbook of memories and photos.
- Create ancestor rituals (e.g., sprinkle rose petals around the pictures of deceased relatives as a part of other ceremonies, e.g., weddings).
- Plant a strong, healthy tree or rose bush in a loved one's name.
- Create a memorial garden and add a new plant on an anniversary.
- Find a tree and tie a yellow ribbon around it. Go there to remember. This is especially helpful when ashes have been scattered and there is no grave.
- Offering a scholarship in a loved one's name.
- On birthdays, holidays, and anniversaries, buy a gift in memory of your loved one, and donate it to someone in need.
- During special religious times of the year, bring up a special item in remembrance of your loved one.
- Have wedding ring made into a new setting (e.g., a necklace, bracelet, etc.).
- Have a birthday celebration for your loved one, and invite guests to wear the deceased's favorite color, and enjoy his or her favorite food.
- Have a family *memory* evening, where you share pictures, reminisce about special times, create a scrapbook of memories, etc.

Special considerations for children and adolescents

 Risk factors for complicated grief in children or adolescents

According to Worden (1996), there are a number of factors that render a bereaved child vulnerable to increased difficulties:

- Sudden deaths, suicides, homicides.
- Death of a mother, for girls before, or in, early adolescence.
- Death of father, for pre-teen and adolescent boys.
- Stigma associated with, or media focus on, suicide or homicide.
- Conflictual relationship with deceased person prior to death.
- Lack of reality; unable to spend time with deceased person after death.
- Inadequate preparation for funeral.
- Pre-existing psychological difficulties.
- Psychologically vulnerable parent (e.g., dependent on child, drugs/alcohol).
- Lack of family and community support.
- Unstable environment (e.g., disruption of routine, inappropriate discipline).
- Poor family coping (e.g., lack of open communication, poor problem-solving).
- Immediate dating by surviving parent.
- Remarriage of surviving parent, if child's relationship with stepparent is negative.

The more risk factors present, the greater difficulty the child will have coping with the death. [23] The child and family should be referred for specialized bereavement counseling. For resources for children, call your local hospice or family and children's services.

No act of kindness, no matter how small, is ever wasted.
Aesop

I don't know what to say to the grieving

The best way to help a grieving person is by reaching out and making contact, and being physically and emotionally present. Don't allow your own sense of helplessness to keep you from reaching out. Understand that everyone grieves in their own way and you cannot take away their pain, but you can be a supportive part of their life.

Do not wait for them to call or contact you, as they may not have the energy or motivation to call, and they may not want to burden you. [49]

You may be wondering how you can be supportive of someone who is grieving. It is important to understand the circumstances of their loss, as each death will be mourned differently.

For example:

The age of the person may have relevance; grieving may be different when an elderly person dies than when a child dies.

The circumstances of the death may have relevance; if the death was sudden, or because of an accident, homicide, or suicide, grieving maybe different than the death of someone with a long illness.

The closeness of the relationship to the person will have an impact on grieving. [56]

Early on, it may be more important just to be present and listen, as there may be no words to help take away the pain. If you act from a place of love and compassion, you will find the words. Remember that it's never too late to call or visit, and offer your assistance and support.

Allow for tears and laughter by saying:
    "It's okay to cry."
    "It's okay to laugh."

Don't try to take the pain away.

Don't rush the grieving process.

Spend time and listen.

Some samples of simple, compassionate things you can say to those grieving the loss of a loved one:

"I am sorry for your loss."

"I am thinking of you at this difficult time."

"I am remembering —— and treasuring my experience with—-."

"The world is a richer place for—— having been here."

"May you find your way to some peace with your loss." [56]

Phrases That Do Help
Door openers:
- "This must be very painful for you."
- "You must have been very close to him."
- "I have no idea of what it must be like for you; I've never had a (spouse/child /parent) die. Can you tell me what it's like?"
- "It must be hard to accept."
- "I really miss ——. He was a special person. But my missing him can't compare with how much you must miss him. Tell me what it's like?" [52]

Phrases that don't help
- "She isn't hurting anymore."
- "It must have been his time."
- "Time will heal."

- "It was God's will."
- "I know how you feel; be thankful you have another child."
- "There must have been a reason." [52]

How often we underestimate the power of a touch, a smile, a kind word. All of which have the potential to turn a life around.
Leo Buscaglia

Special considerations for children and adolescents

 Supporting children after loss

According to Charles Smith, there are four keys to helping children come to terms with a loss: information; emotional expression; tenderness; and reminiscing. Below are some examples of how to speak to children. It is important to consider the child's age and abilities, and their previous experience with loss. You should offer opportunities for children to ask questions and to express their feelings.

- **Tell the child about the loss in a clear language.**
- **Help children learn about loss, grief, and death.**
- **Encourage play.**
- **Protect the child's need for privacy.**

- **Listen to their feelings and their concerns.**
- **Encourage their release of feelings.**
- **Maintain their regular daily activities and routines.**
- **Provide opportunity to remember the loved one.**
- **Show affection when appropriate. [75]**

The grieving of children may be expressed differently from adults. Children, of all ages, experience a sense of sadness, loss, and pain, with common themes, including fear of death and being left alone. There may be feelings of guilt, and concern that the other parent will die too. [16]

Moving on, giving back, life after death

Grief cannot be bypassed; it must be experienced. Healing takes time, and it can be overwhelming at times. The process of mourning is similar to the process of healing. After healing has occurred, it's okay to move on, even though there will still be a scar left. You may find you have the opportunity to do and try new things, make new friends, join new groups, and develop new interests. [48] You will find that as you have survived, the pain does lessen, and healing does occur. Letting go and forgiving the other person, as well as yourself, and possibly God, will allow you to feel lighter as you go forward. You may find now you can be kind to yourself by not neglecting your own emotional and medical well-being. You should be able to focus on nutrition, exercise, meditation, prayer, and positive things that you enjoy, going forward.

If you find your mood continues to be low, or depression is lasting longer than expected, you should seek medical help with your family practitioner, as depression may need to be treated. This is a time to be kind to yourself, love yourself, and care for yourself. Now is the time to come to terms with living your life without your loved one. Over the next several months, it will be important for you to maintain contact with your support system, friends, family, and counselors, as this may be a time when you may feel loneliness and sadness, especially around special dates and holidays. You may need to adjust to new roles in your life, and a reorganization may be a welcome change.

You have not lived today until you have done something for someone who can never repay you.
John Bunyan

Some people find that, as part of their healing and moving on, they are inspired to give back by helping others through their own grief process. There are opportunities to volunteer with peer grief counseling, through places like hospice and other community services.

Anne is a retired registered nurse, and an author, who works as a volunteer for Hospice Niagara in many different capacities. She works as a visiting volunteer; at day hospice, and she provides reiki treatments. I asked her how it was she became a volunteer at hospice. She expressed that she had worked in a variety of volunteer positions in the past. She began volunteering at Hospice Niagara when it first opened, over ten years ago. She asserts that, "Volunteering has helped me to overcome some of the anxieties that I have in my own life." Anne is the author of three books. She started using journaling as a way to release her anxiety and emotions, and out of that came her first book, *I love You Letters from a Loving Friend*. She continued with her book, *I Hear You Responses from a Loving Friend,* and her third book, *God Glasses,* has also been published. She states her work with hospice enables her to have some self-reflection. Her own story includes the illness of her husband, Bert. She had been volunteering at hospice before he became sick. She states, "I had a phenomenal experience at Hospice Niagara, the Stabler Centre, when Bert was dying. I felt that when he was admitted to the inpatient hospice, I was released from prison; I didn't feel alone in his care. After five weeks in the residential hospice, Bert looked at me and said, 'I haven't got the energy to go on.' I said, 'Love, let go,' and two days later, he died." After the death of her husband, Anne continues to volunteer at hospice. She declares, "My faith in God has allowed me to move on and to give back."

If you are interested in volunteering, contact your local hospice, or visit the grief/healing websites listed on my website, **www.HomeHospiceBook.com,** to find a community volunteer service near you.

---

*Let us touch the dying, the poor, the lonely, and the unwanted,
according to the graces we have received, and let us not be
ashamed or slow to do the humble work.*
Mother Teresa

My notes, thoughts, and questions

I highly recommend that you write down any ideas, questions, thoughts, and reflections that may be important to you. Please feel free to use your book as a companion on this, your journey, and take your book with questions to your care providers to help start those difficult conversations.

This final chapter in *The Book of Home Hospice* has covered the topics of grief and bereavement. As you move forward, it's important to understand that your grief will ebb and flow like the tides; there will be times when you feel better, and times when you feel sad, and cry. Always remember, you are not alone, and you can reach out in those times.

Finally, if you have been inspired by this book, please pass it along to someone in need.

To purchase more copies, visit my website at **www.HomeHospiceBook.com, or www.amazon.com.**

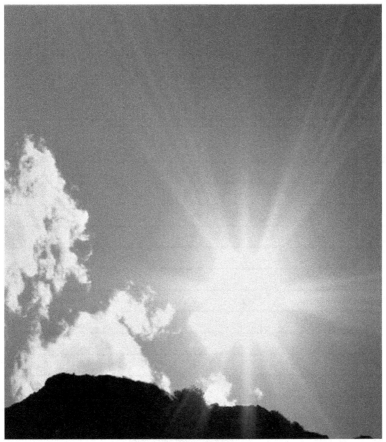

Photo.credit:Johnathon.Dooler2017

Notes

About the Author

Deborah Dooler, MD CCFP (PC), is a physician specializing in palliative care with the South Niagara Palliative Care Outreach Team, an Assistant Clinical Professor at the McMaster University Michael DeGroote Medical School, and a member of the faculties of family and palliative medicine at McMaster University.

She was educated as a registered nurse at Niagara College Mac School of Nursing, graduating in 1997. She continued her education at Brock University, gaining a BA in Community Health Science, while working as an intensive care nurse and raising her three children. She finished her Medical Degree in 2005, from McMaster University Michael DeGroote School of Medicine, and completed her family medicine postgraduate residency at McMaster University in Hamilton, Ontario, Canada, in 2007.

She has been a professor at McMaster University Michael DeGroote School of Medicine, Niagara Campus, since its inaugural year in 2008. She continues to enjoy teaching and mentoring medical students, clinical clerks, and residents, while encouraging them to consider the great rewards and benefits of doing home visits.

After graduating family medicine residency, she began working as an acute care hospitalist with the Niagara Health System. During her time working in the hospital, she began a focused practice of palliative care, looking after the dying. She worked as the Chief of Hospital Medicine, for the Niagara Health System, and was a member of the Executive Team. In 2013, she became the founding Medical Director for the South Niagara Palliative Outreach Team, where she continues to practice today.

Deborah is the Founder and CEO of The Dooler Institute. She enjoys spreading her knowledge and wisdom in the areas of end-of-life care and mindfulness. Her motto is, "Be happy, be grateful, and see the silver linings," encouraging people to live their life until there is no more life to live. She lives in Fenwick, Ontario, with her husband, John, and loves spending time with her adult children, Rick, Amy, and Johnathon.

The author is available for delivering presentations and workshops. For rates and availability, please contact the author directly at: **drdooler@homehospicebook.com.**

To order more books, please visit: www.HomeHospice Book.com, or www.amazon.com.

Back cover photo credit: Stephen Franklin Photography, Fenwick, Ontario.

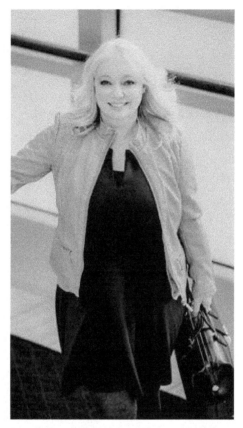

Photo.credit:Stephen.Franklin2015

Citations

1. Gomes et al. *BMC Palliative Care* 2013, 12:7 http://www.biomedcentral.com/1472-684X/12/7

2. Sandsdalen et al. *BMC Palliative Care* (2016) 15:79 DOI 10.1186/s12904-016-0152-1

3. Ruijs et al. *BMC Family Practice* 2013, 14:201 http://www.biomedcentral.com/1471-2296/14/201

4. Canadian Hospice Palliative Care Association. *A Model to Guide Hospice Palliative Care.* Ottawa, Canadian Hospice Palliative Care Association, 2015.

5. http://www.chpca.net/professionals/ethics.aspx

6. https://www.cma.ca/Assets/assets-library/document/en/advocacy/cma_policy_advance_care_planning_pd15-08-e.pdf

7. http://www.cpso.on.ca/CPSO/media/documents/Policies/Policy-Items/End-of-Life.pdf?ext=.pdf

8. Amery, Justin. *Children's Palliative for Doctors and Nurses Anywhere in the World.* New York, Lulu Publishing, 2016.

9. Marty Hogan. *If I Should Die... the Dying Process: What to Expect and Things You Can Do to Help.* New York, Sacred vigil press, 2007.

10. Pallium Canada. *The Pallium Palliative Pocketbook.* Ottawa, Pallium Canada, 2016.

11. Pallium Canada. *Learning Essential Approaches to Palliative and End-of-Life Care.* Ottawa, Pallium Canada, 2016.

12. http://www.dyingmatters.org/page/interesting-facts-about-dying

13. http://canyouactually.com/23-strange-and-disturbing-facts-about-death-that-will-surprise-you/

14. Palliative Pain and Symptom Management Consultation Program. *The Fundamentals of Hospice Palliative Care: A Resource Guide for Formal Caregivers.* Straffordville, Sportswood Printing, 2012.

15. Harry van Bommel. *Saint Elizabeth Healthcare Foundation Family Hospice Care Pre-planning and Care Guide.* Scarborough, Webcom, Ltd, 2002.

16. Macmillan, Karen. *A Caregiver's Guide: A Handbook About End of Life.* Edmonton, Palliative Care Association of Alberta, 2000.

17. Elizabeth Kubler-Ross. *Questions and Answers on Death and Dying.* New York, Macmillan Publishing Company, 1974.

18. Elizabeth Kubler-Ross. *On Death and Dying: What the Dying Have to Teach Doctors, Nurses, Clergy, and Their Own Families.* New York, Macmillan Publishing Company, 1969.

19. http://www.dyingconsciously.org/history.html

20. http://www.chpca.net/media/319547/norms-of-practice-eng-web.pdf

21. http://hospice.org.nz/cms_show_download.php?id=854

22. https://www.ipc.on.ca/wp-content/uploads/Resources/circle-of-care.pdf

23. Liana Lowenstein. *Creative Interventions for Bereaved Children.* Toronto, Champion Press, 2006.

24. Elizabeth J Latimer. *Miles to Go: A Handbook of Comfort and Support for People Who are Seriously Ill.* Toronto, Prentice-Hall, 1998.

25. Elizabeth J Latimer. *Easing the Hurt: A Handbook of Comfort for Families and Friends of People Who are Seriously Ill.* Toronto, Prentice-Hall, 1998.

26. Canadian Hospice Palliative Care Association. *A guide for Caregivers.* Ottawa, 2015.

27. Mervyn Dean. *Symptom Relief in Palliative Care.* Oxon, Radcliffe Publishing Ltd, 2011.

28. http://www.mayoclinic.org/diseases-conditions/bed-sores/manage/ptc-20315637

29. *Sexuality in Cancer and Palliative Care 1: Effects of Disease and Treatment.* https://www.ncbi.nlm.nih.gov/ pubmed/12411851

30. *Providing Urinary Continence Care to Adults at the End of Life.* https://www.nursingtimes.net/clinical-archive/ continence/providing-urinary-continence-care-to-adults-at-the-end-of-life/5004035.article

31. *Intimacy Issues in Palliative Care: How to Ask.* http://www.medscape.com/viewarticle/873525

32. *Sexuality and Intimacy Within the Context of Life-Threatening Illness: Implications for Hospice and Palliative Care Professionals.*
https://www.nhpco.org/sexuality-and-intimacy-within-context-life-threatening-illness-implications-hospice

33. *The Prevalence, Key Causes and Management of Insomnia in Palliative Care Patients.* http://www.jpsmjournal.com/article/S0885-3924(04)00009-0/abstract

34. Goldstein and Morrison. *Evidence Based Practice of Palliative Medicine.* Philadelphia, Elsevier, 2013.

35. http://kokuamau.org/resources/last-stages-life

36. http://www.virtualhospice.ca

37. https://medicalmarijuana.ca/patients/marijuana-laws/

38. https://wwhttp://www.hamiltonhealthsciences.ca/workfiles/Palliative%20Care/MAIDFAQ.pdfw.cannimed.ca/pages/thc-and-cbd

39. http://www.endoflifeadvisor.com/how-to-forgive/

40. Alan D. Wolfelt. *Creating Meaningful Funeral Ceremonies: A Guide for Caregivers.* Fort Collins, Companion Press, 1994.

41. https://en.wikipedia.org

42. http://www.aberdeenfuneralhome.com/memorial-services

43. https://www.mcscs.jus.gov.on.ca/english/DeathInvestigations/WholeBodyDonation/DI_body_donation.html

44. https://www.ontario.ca/page/what-do-when-someone-dies#section-0

45. http://www.investopedia.com/articles/personal-finance/121914/life-insurance-policies-how-payouts-work.asp

46. http://www.rcmp-grc.gc.ca/cfp-pcaf/fs-fd/will-testament-eng.htm

47. John D. Martin and Frank D. Ferris. *I Can't Stop Crying: It's So Hard When Someone You Love Dies.* Toronto, Key Porter Books, 1992.

48. Melba Colgrave, Harold Bloomfield, Peter McWilliams. *How to Survive the Loss of a Love.* Los Angeles, Prelude Press, 1991.

49. Therese Rando. *Grief, Dying, and Death: Clinical Interventions for Caregivers.* Champaign, Research Press Company, 1984.

50. Judith McCoyd, Carolyn Walter. *Grief and Loss Across the Lifespan: A Biopsychosocial Perspective.* New York, Springer Publishing Company, 2016.

51. Rose Caelin. *Bereavement Risk Assessment Tool Brat Manual.* Victoria, Victoria Hospice Society, 2007.

52. Kelly Osmont, Marilyn McFarlane. *What Can I Say? How to Help Someone Who is Grieving: A Guide.* Portland, Nobility Press, 1988.

53. Bill Webster. *Now what?* Mississauga, Centre for the Grief Journey, 1995.

54. J William Worden. *Grief Counseling and Grief Therapy: A Handbook for the Mental Health Practitioner.* New York, Springer Publishing Company, 2002.

55. Katherine Ashenburg. *The Mourners Dance: What We Do When People Die.* Toronto, Macfarlane Walter and Ross, 2002.

56. Susan P Halpern. *The Etiquette of Illness: What to Say When You Can't Find the Words.* New York, Bloomsbury, 2004.

57. Laurie Lemieux, Stefanie Kaiser, Jose Pereira, Lynn Meadows. *Sexuality in Palliative Care: Patient Perspectives.* https://www.ncbi.nlm.nih.gov/pubmed/15540672.

58. Frank Ostaseski. *The Five Invitations: Discovering What Death Can Teach Us About Living Fully.* New York, Flatiron Books, 2017.

59. Jon Kabat-Zinn. *Wherever You Go, There You Are: Mindfulness Meditation in Everyday Life.* New York, Hyperion,

2017.

60. Philip Kapleau. *The Zen of Living and Dying: A Practical and Spiritual Guide.* Boston, Shambhala, 1998.

61. Doreen Virtue and James Van Praagh. *How to Heal a Grieving Heart.* New York, Hay House Inc., 2013.

62. Rhonda Byrne. *The Secret.* New York, Beyond Words, 2006.

63. Emma Seppala. *That Happiness Track.* New York, Harper Collins, 2016.

64. *Complementary and Alternative Medicine in Cancer Pain Management: A Systematic Review.*
https://www.ncbi.nlm.nih.gov/pmc/articles/PMC4332115/

65. *Factors Important to Patients' Quality of Life at the End of Life.*
https://www.ncbi.nlm.nih.gov/pmc/articles/PMC3806298/

66. Alesha Gaudet. *Best Practice Guidelines for Multi-Sensory Stimulation Therapy: A Palliative Care Intervention.* St. Johns, Canadian Palliative Care Association, 2011.

67. Alesha Gaudet, Mary Lou Stephens, Shelly Tallon, Kathy Cameau, Jackie McDonald, Lina Moore, Stephan Bilynsky, Anna Grenier, Loretta Turpin, and Donna Pringle. *Quality Palliative Care in Long-Term Snozelen Training Tool Kit.* St. Johns, Canadian Palliative Care Association, 2011.

68. Room 217: Care Through Music. *Music Care Resources Programs and Services.* www.room217.ca

69. *Music Care: Training Caregivers in the Therapeutic Use of Music.* www.musiccareconference.ca

70. http://www.cancer.ca/en/cancer-information/diagnosis-and-treatment/complementary-therapi

es/choosing-a-complementary-therapy-and-practitioner/?region=on

71. http://www.webmd.com/digestive-disorders/tc/dyspepsia-topic-overview

72. https://wellspring.ca/

73. https://www.mindful.org/meditation/mindfulness-getting-started/

74. https://www.ecowatch.com/6-ways-to-deepen-your-spiritual-relationship-to-nature-1881983638.html

75. https://www.takingcharge.csh.umn.edu/explore-healing-practices/healing-environment/what-are-healing-gardens

76. http://pallium.ca/cc/

75. Donna O'Toole, Jerre Cory. *Helping Children Grieve and Grow: A Guide for Those Who Care.* Burnsville, Compassion Books Inc., 2005.

76 Jake Swearingen, *You Should Know Your Parents' Social Media End-of-Life Wishes.* The Atlantic, 2015.

CPSIA information can be obtained
at www.ICGtesting.com
Printed in the USA
LVHW01s1458100918
589690LV00012B/986/P